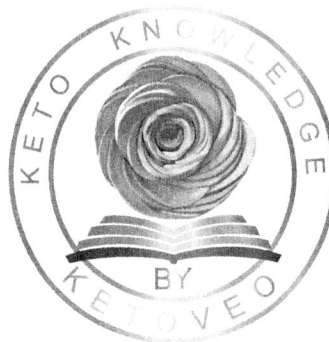

Go to **www.ketoveo.com** for more guides and resources to help you on your keto journey.

CONTENTS

INTRODUCTION

If you are eating a high-carbohydrate diet, you are most likely eating a lot of processed food and high doses of sugar. In doing so, you are not giving your body the nutrients it needs. Instead, you are adding up the calories and potentially increasing your risk of disease. So, what is the solution?

The moment you type the letter 'k' in a Google search, 8 times out of 10, the Ketogenic Diet (or simply Keto Diet) would show up as a search result. What is the Keto Diet? Is it one of those diets which is just an old book with a new cover? Is it an over-blown fad which no one has ever really completed but yet everyone can't stop singing its praises? In a world ruled by buzzwords, is it one of those hyped up diets which one random celebrity came up with and now everyone is doing it?

The answer to all these questions is - no.
First and foremost, the Keto Diet is one of the few diets known which is based on actual solid science. The word 'Keto' is derived from the word ketosis which is the state that the human body goes into where instead of burning carbohydrates (starches and sugars) to generate energy, your body burns stored fat.

Your marvelous human body can use both carbohydrates and fat as the source of energy. But it's inclined to use carbohydrates as the primary source. The main goal of the Keto Diet is to break away from this process and get your body to use fat as its primary fuel.

But how does your body do that?

Well, it needs a little help from you. If you decreased or removed carbohydrates from your diet, your body would have no choice but to shift over to the alternative source. It would begin to consume the stored fat.

But this brings another question, why are carbohydrates the villain here? Let's talk about it first. When you eat high-carb food, it breaks down into glucose before being absorbed into the bloodstream. From this point on, it enters your body cells with the help of insulin. Glucose is used by your body for energy and any unused glucose is converted into glycogen. When more glucose is consumed than that which can be stored as glycogen, it converts to fat. So, now we can see, more carbs means more glucose, more glucose means more fat, and more fat means weight gain.

Imagine, if you had two sources of energy and using one of them causes more harm than good, and then you find out that using the second one will not only provide you enough energy, it will also make you stronger and more fit. This is what the Keto Diet does for your body.

Low-carb intake drives your body to go into a state of ketosis. During ketosis your body is trained to use fat as the main source of energy instead of carbs. Your liver plays an important role in ketosis. When it realizes that there is not enough fuel in the form of carbs to power your body, it breaks down fat into ketones, which in turn allows your body to use fat as energy. You don't stop eating food, you just stop eating carbohydrate-rich food. This process, in tandem with a good workout routine, makes weight loss a walk in the park. And it just doesn't stop at weight loss, it helps you control and fight a lot of other diseases as well.

As with all things that provide great results, "going Keto" comes with an equal amount of hard work. For someone with a sweet-tooth, it is indeed going to be tricky to avoid sugar. But as the saying goes "If it was easy, everyone would have done it." In the end, you'll realize that it was worth the price because you'll feel more fit both physically and mentally.

What is a Ketogenic Diet?

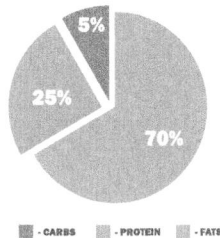

The Ketogenic Diet is the process of manipulating your body to switch its energy source from carbohydrates to the fat which has been stored in your body or which you eat. You do this by controlling the ratio of carbs, fats, and proteins which you consume.

As mentioned earlier, excess fat is the reason we keep adding pounds. In a typical diet, the focus is on working out and then keeping a close eye on the number of calories being consumed. On top of that, you need to make sure that the quantity of calories you burn is always greater than the calorie intake. Because so many variables are involved, it gets difficult which is why people stop following their diet and go back to gaining weight.

A Ketogenic Diet is not only about weight loss. It also helps to control the glucose, or blood sugar in your body. Too much sugar in your body forces the pancreas to work harder to pump out more insulin.

As with any machine, if you keep pushing it to the limit, there comes a point when it will break or stop working at its maximum efficiency. Without enough insulin, the sugar concentration in the blood keeps getting higher and higher and leads to the disease called diabetes. And with diabetes comes high blood pressure, heart disease, kidney disease, and many other maladies.

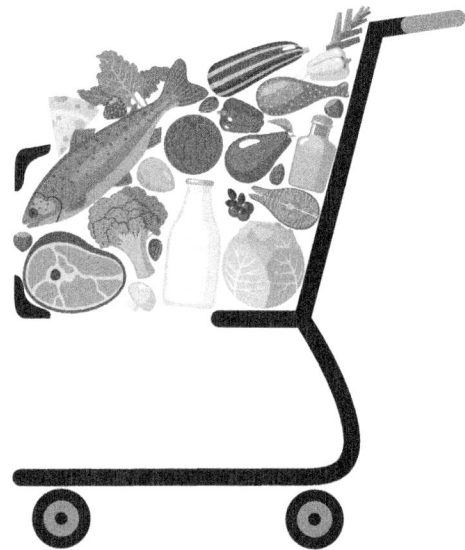

KETOGENIC FOOD

In the Ketogenic Diet we simply need to keep in mind that this is a low-carb, moderate protein, and high fat diet. Compose your daily meals to be 5% carbs, 25% proteins and 70% Fat.

The crucial manipulation of carbs, fats, and protein in a Ketogenic Diet leads to ketosis and you know the rest of the story now.

To state it simply, a Ketogenic Diet can help you lose much more weight than a low-fat diet and it does it without making you super hungry.

CHAPTER 2

Benefits of the Keto Diet

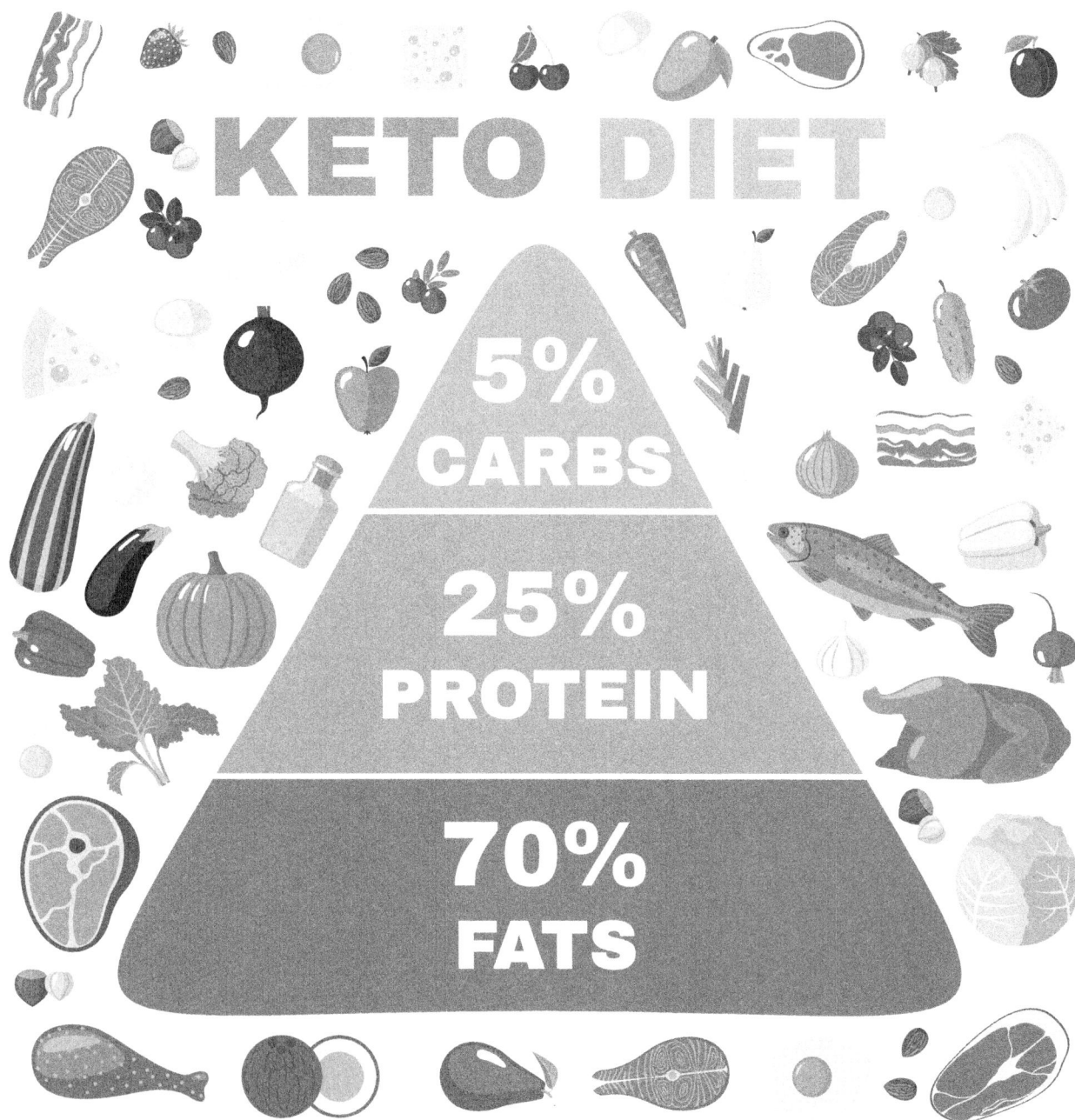

As mentioned earlier the aim of the Ketogenic Diet is to have a daily intake that generally breaks down to consuming 5% carbs maximum, 25% protein and 75% fat.

To work out your daily intake with your health and weight loss goals in mind go to our website Ketoveo.com to use our Macro Calculator which will help you calculate your personal daily intake needs determined by your body weight, height, age and activity levels. This will help you stay on track to get your body into ketosis.

Sugar vs Ketones

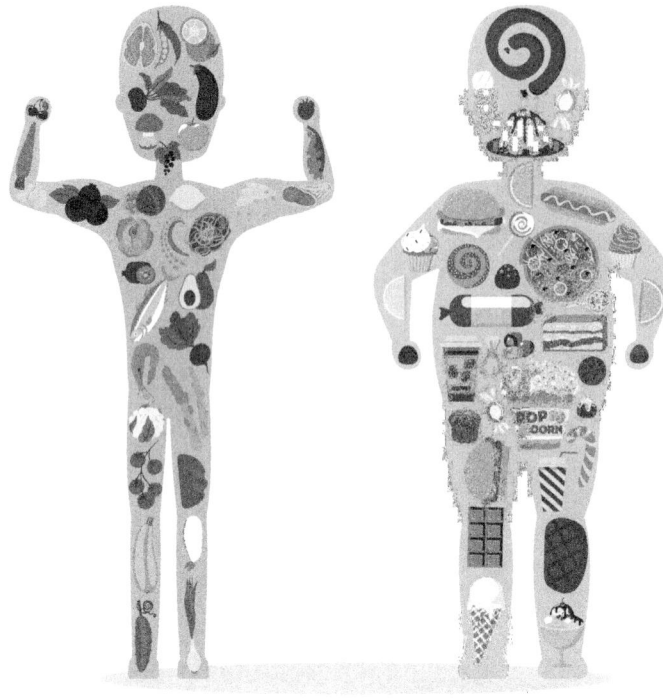

So far, what we are sure of is that the Keto Diet is basically the replacement of carbs by fats as the main source of energy. This, as mentioned before, is the condition called ketosis. The actual fuel being used during ketosis is called ketones. These ketones and sugar do basically the same thing, but how they affect your body cannot be more different. Let's compare the two.

When you eat food, you increase the number of free radicals in your body. Free radicals are types of oxygen-containing molecules which strongly interact with other molecules. But not in a good way. These reactions cause damage to your cells, protein and DNA.

Usually, these free radicals are kept in check by antioxidants. Your body makes some of the antioxidants it needs and some you get from the food you eat. In theory, you have enough antioxidants operating and your body keeps on its merry way to stay healthy. But with an excessive consumption of sugar/carbs, you get too many free radicals and your body's ability to produce enough antioxidants falls far behind and these free radicals then start damaging your organs and functions of your body .

Additionally, a high intake of simple sugars can make cells, including your brain cells, insulin resistant which could cause brain cells to die. On the other hand, ketones help protect the cells in your body by reducing the production of free radicals in your body . This, in turn, has shown to protect neuron cells in the brain. The healthy cells of your body which are being affected by high doses of sugar are also helped by these ketones. It is done by improving the cell health and protecting it from damaging inflammation.

One thing we all need to understand is that there is more to the Ketogenic Diet than just a rapid weight loss technique. It comes with important medical benefits.

Keto Diet & Diabetes

We have established that by utilizing the Ketogenic Diet, you are able to control the amount of glucose in your blood which will then help you to avoid diabetes or at least to control it. Also, Anyone who knows anything about diabetes would tell you that one of the biggest risks is cataracts. Here again, a Keto Diet could help. With active control over carbs and sugar, it could fight to keep any eye related issues at bay and enjoy better vision.

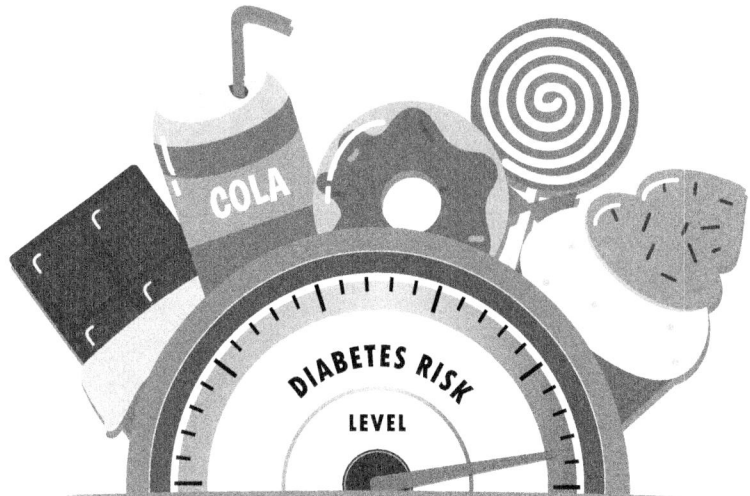

In a recent study, clear signs were found that people with type 2 diabetes are twice as likely to have Alzheimer's than someone who is not a diabetic.

Keto Diet & Alzheimer's Disease

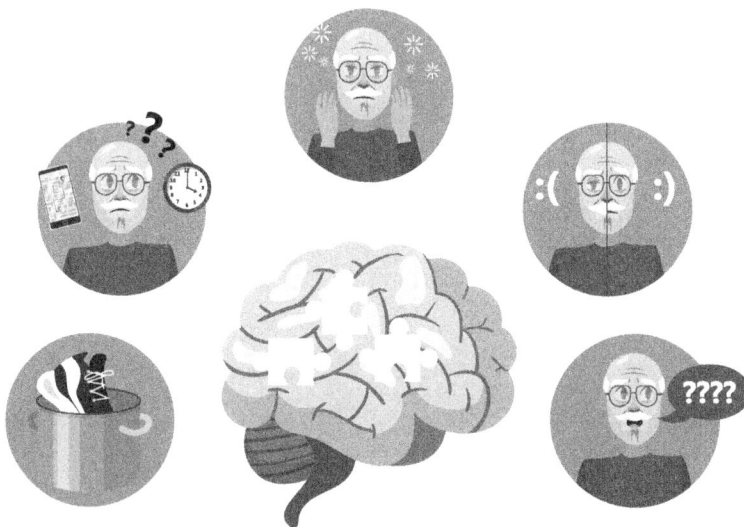

Another study done in 2012 showed that people who ate a high-carb diet had an 80% higher chance of developing mild cognitive impairment. Or in other words, they are on the road to dementia. Although genetic and non-nutritional factors are also responsible for Alzheimer's, more and more people are realizing that food is one factor that can be controlled, and the Ketogenic Diet seems like the best the first step forward.

Since the Ketogenic Diet leads to a healthier and enhanced brain function, it's a wise choice for those seeking a better and healthier brain.

Keto Diet & Fatigue

Do you feel tired on a regular basis? Maybe it's time to look at your diet. If you are on a high-carbohydrate diet, you will feel tired easily. The reason behind this is that carbs are not an efficient source of energy when compared to fats. If you need more efficiency from your body's engine, then you must feed it high-efficiency fuel which (as you must have correctly guessed by now) is fat.

Thus, a Ketogenic Diet can surely put you on the path to becoming the Energizer Bunny of human beings. When you have a more efficient power source, you have a higher output. This holds true for machines as well as humans.

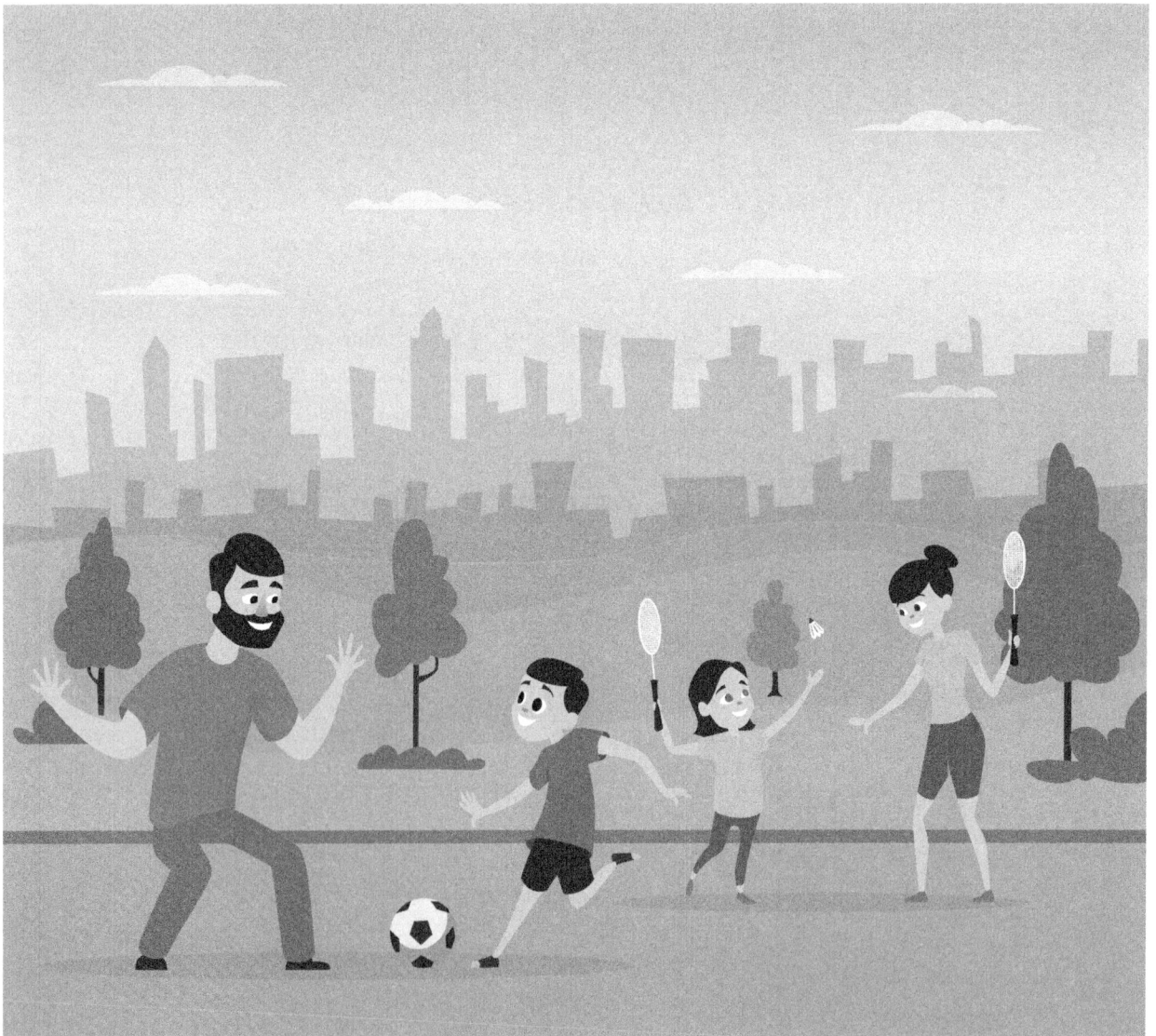

Keto Diet & Acne

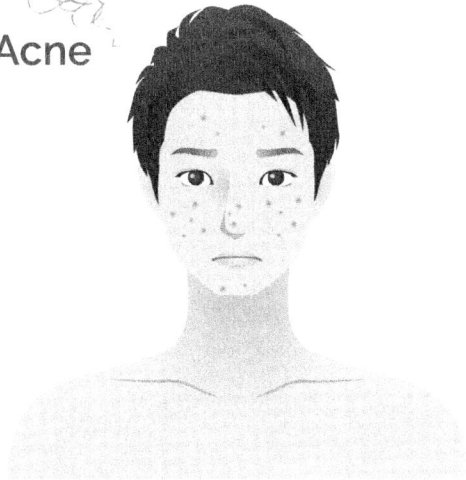

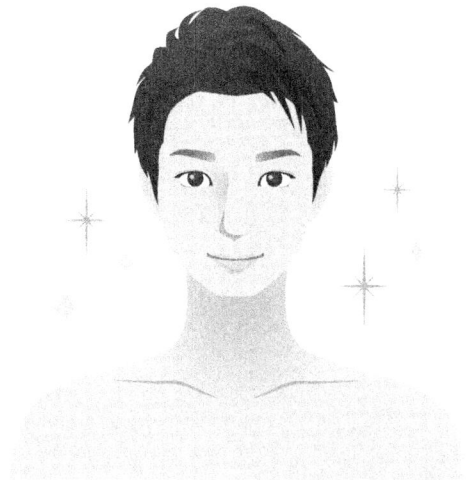

Every time you turn on the TV, you can almost bet that in the first ad break, there will most likely be an ad about acne. You must be wondering why are we talking about acne in a Keto book. Let's dive deeper and see how our favorite villain - carbohydrates - is related to acne and how the Keto Diet can fight that problem.

IGF-1 is a hormone produced by your pituitary gland whose task is to tell your body how many cells to create. Also known as a growth hormone, it controls the rate of creation of new cells and the replacement of the older ones. Under normal circumstances, IGF-1 is needed and does its job well.

However, when the levels of IGF-1 start going over normal, it triggers the creation of a lot of new skin cells. Even though these cells are created beneath the surface of the skin, they slowly rise, and you can guess what happens when they reach the top. There are already cells there and thus begins competition for space and resources. As a result, they end up blocking the pores and they provide the optimal condition for infection, inflammation and the teenager's greatest enemy: acne.

It doesn't stop there. Increased IGF-1 levels mean more sebum. Sebum is an oil naturally produced by your body to keep your skin moisturized and to protect it against bacteria. But excess sebum can lead to blocked pores which in turn leads to acne. So excess IGF-1 starts a chain reaction which can lead to acne.

This brings up the question, what could cause excess IGF-1 to be produced? The answer is: carbohydrates. If you have been eating a high-carb diet and are wondering why you have acne, now you know who the culprit is here.

On the other side is the Ketogenic Diet, where you control the intake of carbohydrates, which implies less glucose and sugar in your body and this, in turn, keeps IGF-1 levels from overflowing. Once this overflow is avoided, the conditions are ripe for you to have an acne free face.

Having too many carbs in your diet is definitely one of the reasons which can cause acne, however, there are others. But the food you eat is something that is completely in your control and if you decide to follow the Ketogenic way, you have a good shot at having clearer, healthier skin.

Keto Diet & Aging

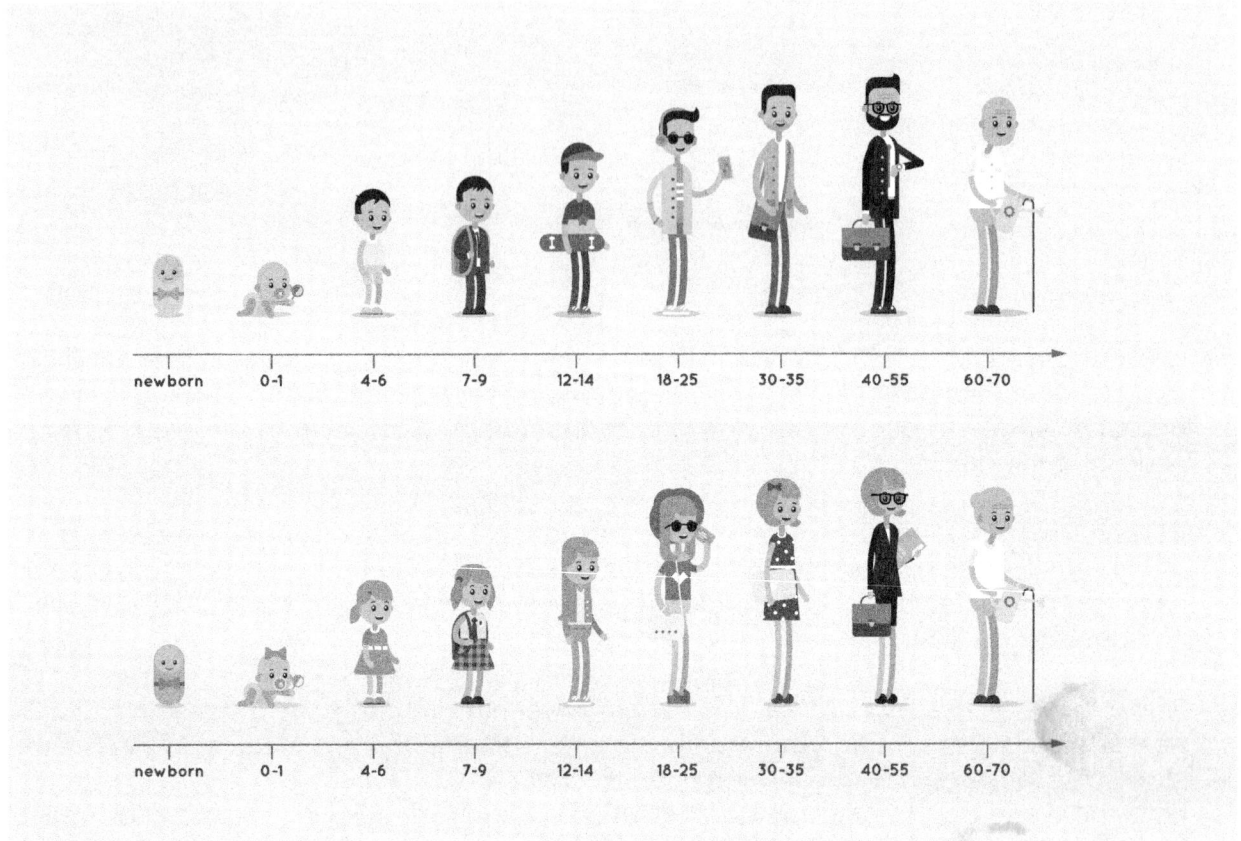

That brings us to the next benefit: the Ketogenic Diet is anti-aging. How? Let's look at the information we have gathered so far.

We all start our human journey from one cell. This cell divides into two and then these two cells split into four and so on and so forth. All these cells combine to form different parts of our body. But there is a limit to how many times each cell can divide, and this limit is called the Hayflick limit. One cell divides approximately fifty times and then it reaches the Hayflick limit, stops dividing and begins to die.

Now think of what we have learned and found earlier in this article: the Ketogenic Diet enhances the health of our cells while sugar degrades them. With the Ketogenic Diet, our cells stay healthy longer and perform better, which in turn means the average lifetime of a cell increases and thus our body is able to stay "younger" for longer which delays the natural aging process.

The Ketogenic Diet enhances the ability of the little power plants in our bodies, called mitochondria, to provide energy in a manner that reduces inflammation and oxidative stress. Although the studies on this have been limited, it makes sense to assume that this diet can help us feeling and looking younger and stronger for longer than the sugar-rich carbohydrate diets that the average person consumes every day.

Keto Diet & Autism

In 2018, a study was published which showed a significant reduction in symptoms for some autistic children on the Ketogenic Diet. It is known that inflammation is an important factor in causing autism. Since the Ketogenic Diet can help control inflammation, it is an effective asset dealing with autistic symptoms.

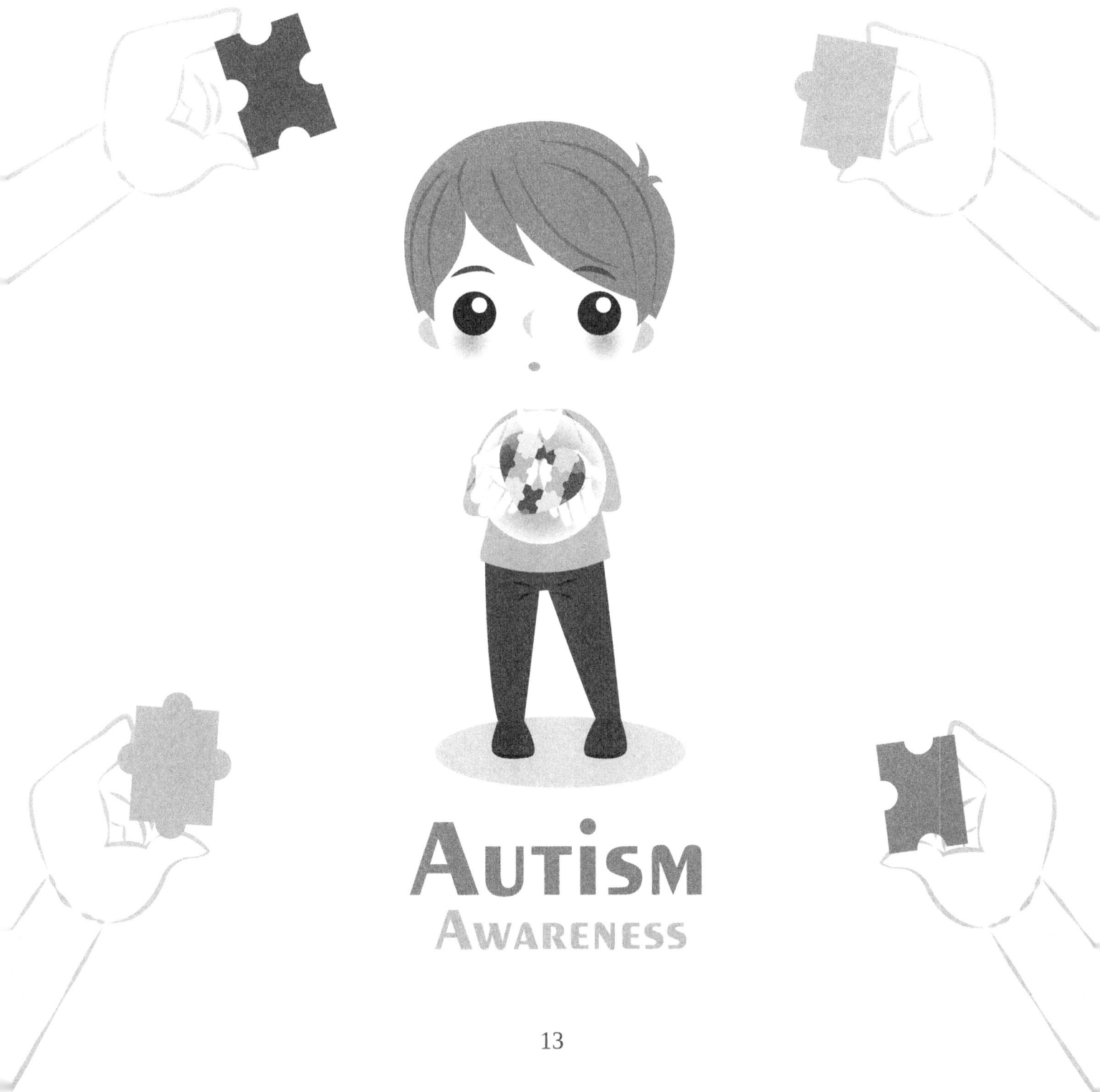

AUTISM
AWARENESS

CHAPTER 3

The Ingredients of a Keto Diet

Most people do not associate fats with being healthy and strong. But after an introduction to the Ketogenic Diet, maybe it's time we stopped looking at fats as an enemy but instead saw them as an ally in our battle against unhealthy living. Let's look at some examples and figure out what exactly a Ketogenic Diet is composed of.

KETO
FOOD BASKET

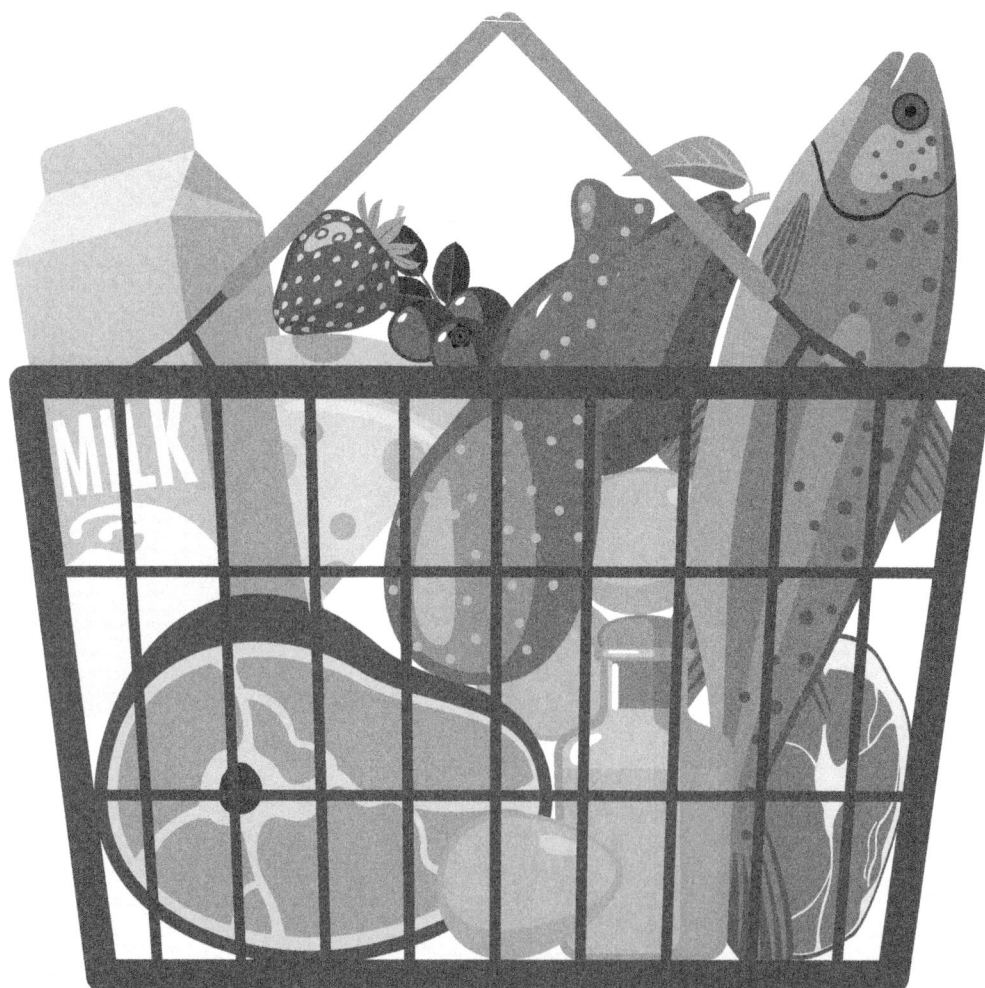

SEA FOOD SET

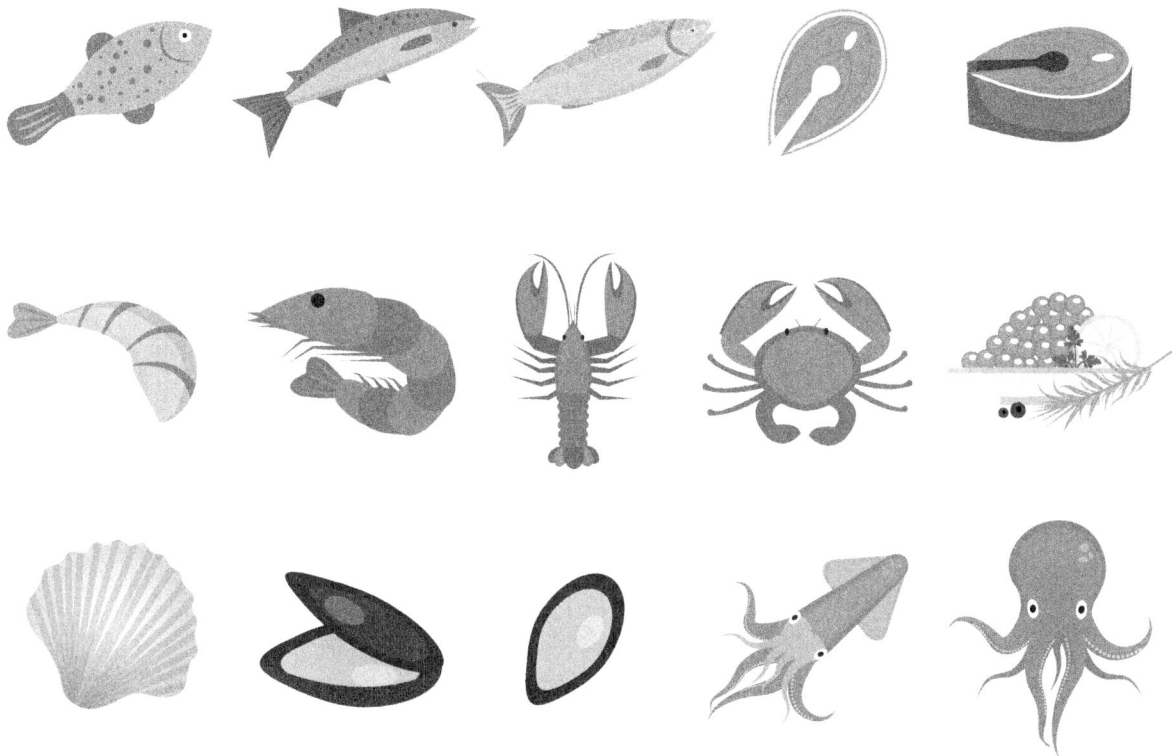

Fish are often called "brain food" because they can provide the necessary nutrition to the brain cells due to the omega-3 and omega-6 fatty acids found in them. The human brain is nearly 60 percent fat. Fatty acids are among the most crucial components that determine your brain's integrity and ability to perform. Since brain tissue primarily consists of fatty acids, any diet that provides these will likely improve your brain.

Salmon and other fish should be one of your main foods. Fish is also high in vitamins and minerals. Best of all, they are virtually carb-free. But keep an eye on the carb content of shellfish. Salmon can easily be the king of the Ketogenic Diet as it not only consists of almost no carbs, it is also very high in omega-3 fatty acids and has been shown to lower insulin levels. It is also known to increase insulin sensitivity in overweight and obese young adults. Eating twice per week should be your target.

VEGETABLES (low-carb vegetables)

If it's green and leafy, gobble it up as soon as you can. It's the best advice you can give to anyone. Many vegetables are very low-carb and filled with almost every possible vitamin and minerals known to mankind.

They have the added advantage that they are full of fiber. Although fiber is technically a carbohydrate, your body cannot fully digest it and therefore it cannot be broken down into sugar molecules. Fiber is great for helping regulate blood sugar and hunger.

Remember the free-radicals we spoke about earlier? Vegetables contain antioxidants which can help protect against free radicals and prevent cell damage. Spinach, brussels sprouts, kale, broccoli, and cauliflower are the best replacements for any high-carb diet.

But not all vegetables will work on a Keto Diet. You will want to steer away from potatoes, yams, corn and other high-starch vegetables as they will turn the tables on your diet very easily and quickly.

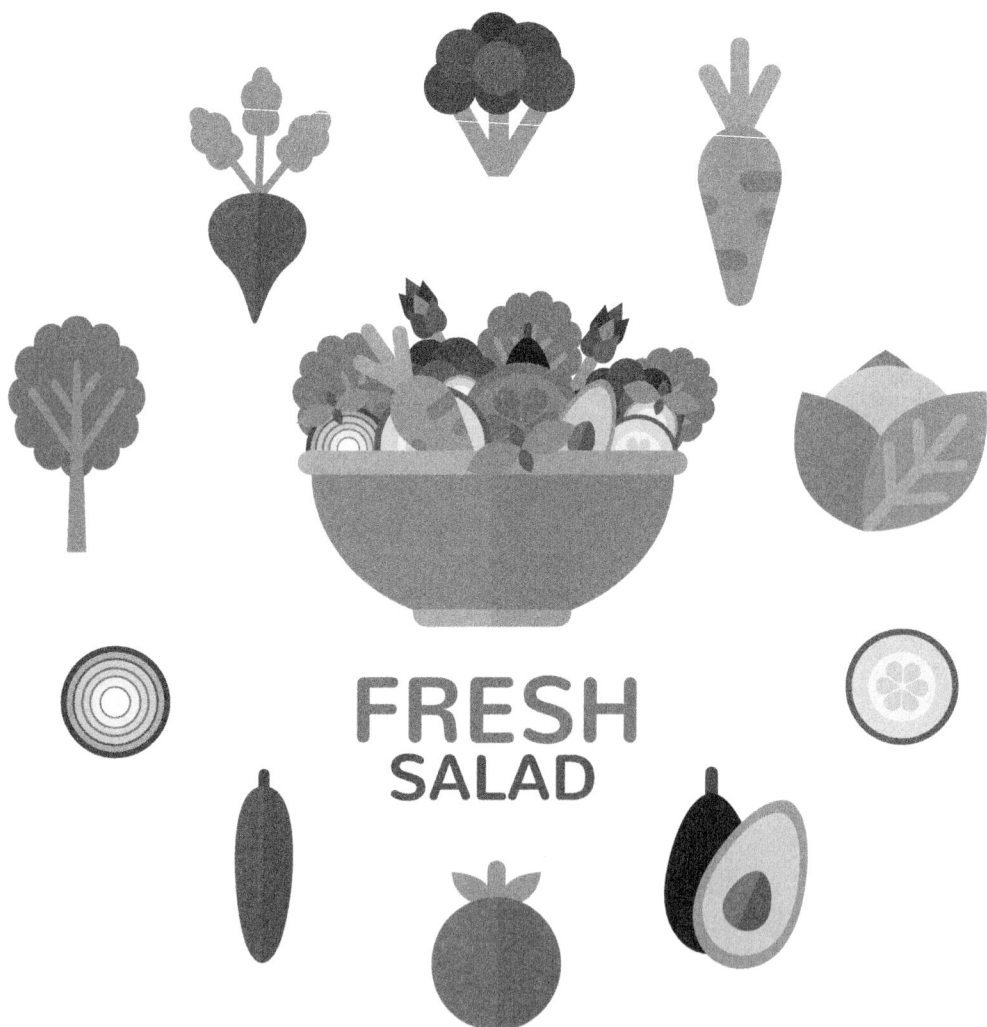

FRESH
SALAD

DAIRY PRODUCTS

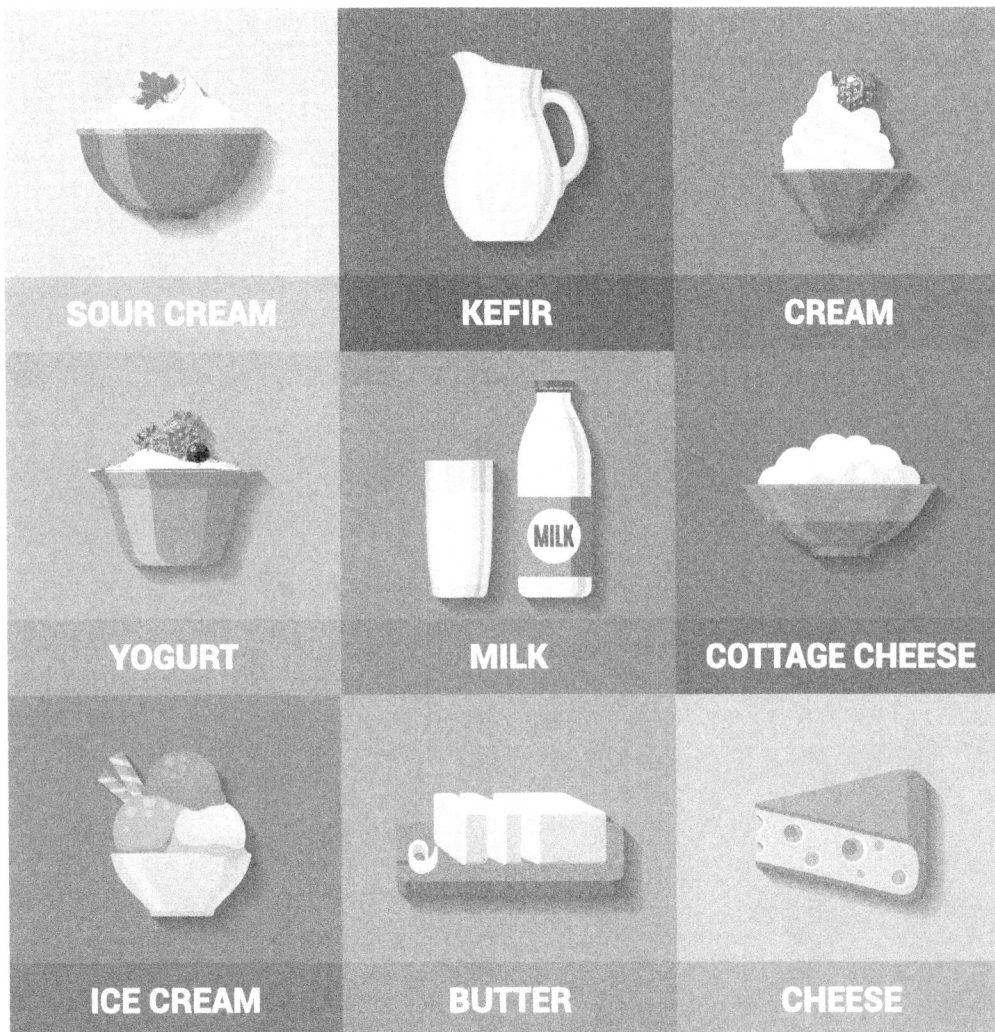

Cheese is something that will not only add to the taste of your Keto Diet, it is also something that will give you a high amount of fat, protein, and calcium.

Yogurt is a wonderful source of protein and calcium. Plain Greek yogurt may have no fat in it, but it has only 7 grams of carbs and a whopping 24 grams of protein in a cup. But remember to stay away from the flavoured ones, they will upturn your Keto cart in one meal. They are a storehouse for sugar. If you want a bit of flavour, add a few berries to the yogurt to satisfy your taste buds.

AVOCADOS

Avocados are the numero uno of the Keto Diet. It is 15% fat, most of which is the type of fat which helps to lower bad cholesterol. As well, avocados have loads of vitamins and minerals. No wonder it is called a superfood.

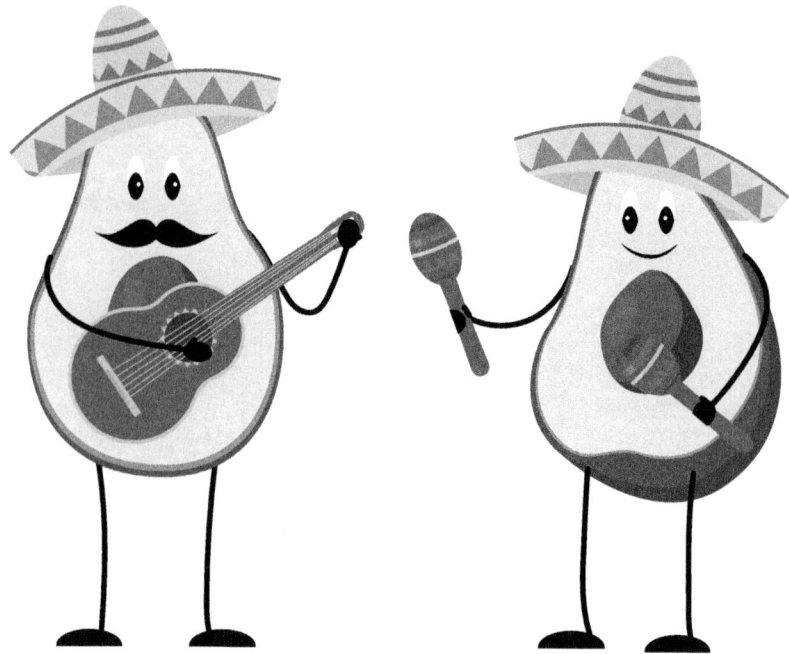

MEAT & POULTRY

Meat and poultry are staples of the Keto Diet. Low on carbs and high on proteins and fat, they can fit into just about any meal. A study that was done on Australian beef found animals that are grass fed produce meat with higher amounts of omega-3 and antioxidants than meat from grain fed animals. Whether it is the chicken thighs or the New York strip steak, they will keep your fat and protein intake in sync with your Keto plan.

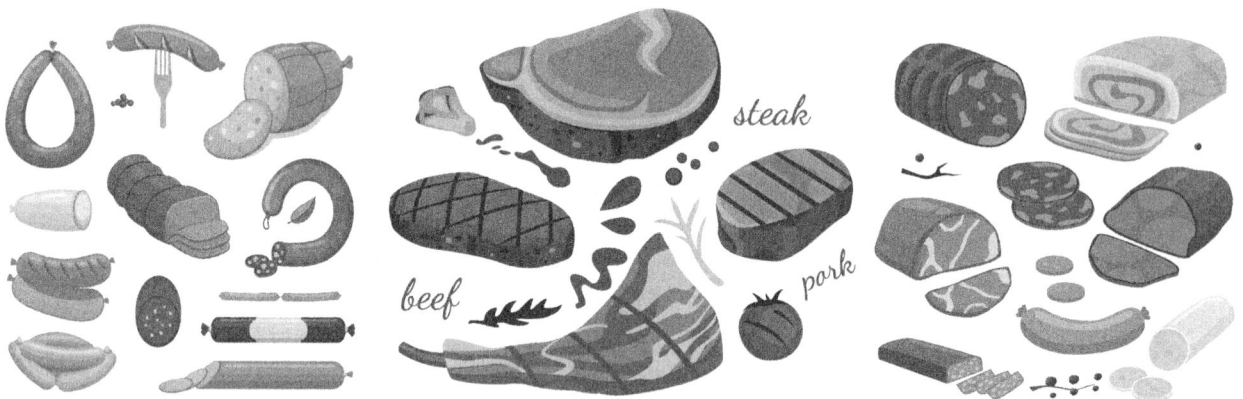

EGGS

Eggs truly are incredible. They are high in protein, high in fat, and very low on carbs. A boiled egg contains around 11 grams of fat, 13 grams of protein, and only 1 gram of carbs. Eggs are one of the most nutrient dense foods on the planet! For most people, eating the yolk doesn't increase the cholesterol in your body very much, but if one is diabetic, it might be best to stay away from the yolk and stick to the egg whites.

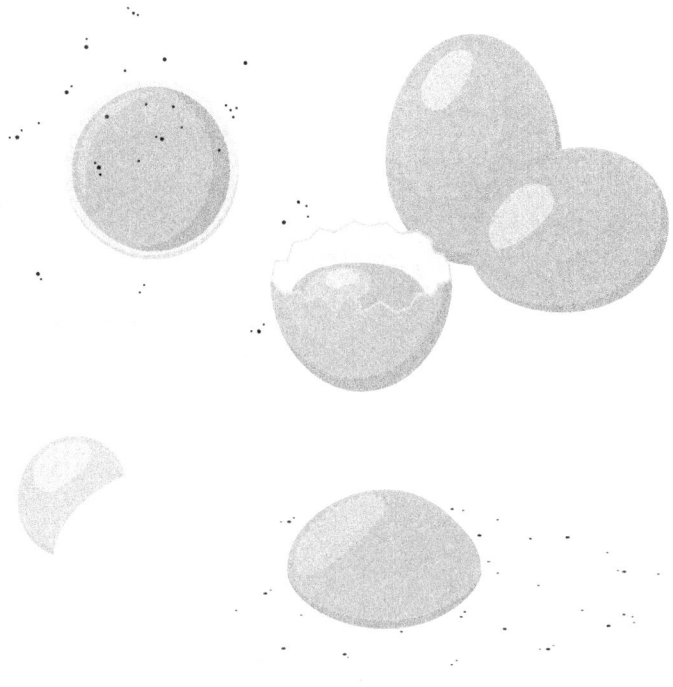

COCONUT OIL

MCT (Medium-chain triglycerides) are found in coconuts and can aid in weight loss. Their specialty is that (unlike the long-chain triglycerides) they metabolize differently and go directly to the liver, where they are turned into ketones.

These ketones are what we need for a successful Ketogenic Diet. These ketones can cross from the blood to the brain and can provide an alternate source of energy for the brain. Moreover, since the calories contained in the MCTs are burnt more efficiently and used by your body , the probability of them being stored as fat is minimal.

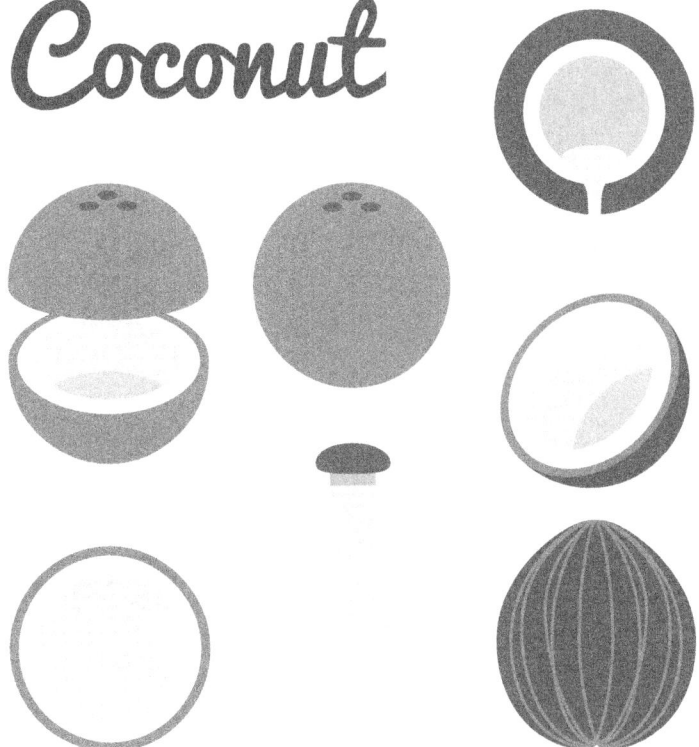

DARK CHOCOLATE/ COCOA POWDER

Considered one of the best sources of antioxidants on the planet, a 70-85% dark chocolate is a great option for dessert on the Keto Diet. Just make sure the chocolate you enjoy is sugar-free. Luckily there are many chocolate bars made today using Erythritol, Stevia or other non-sugar sweeteners.

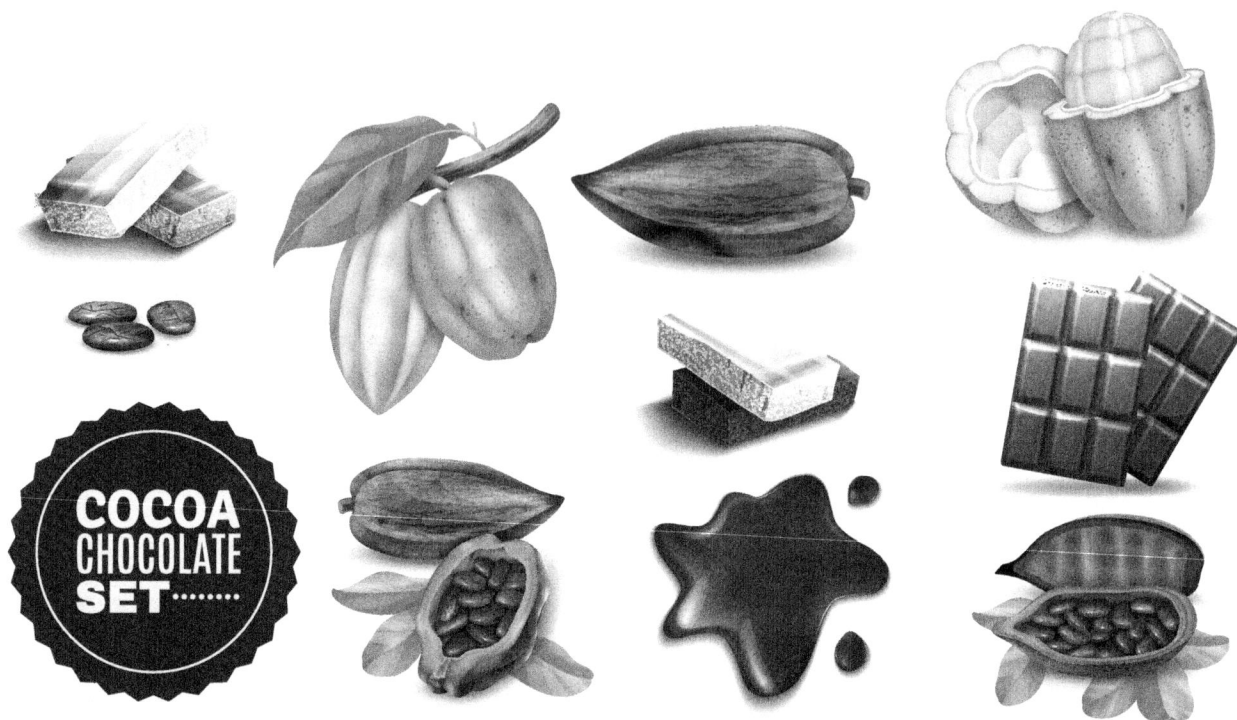

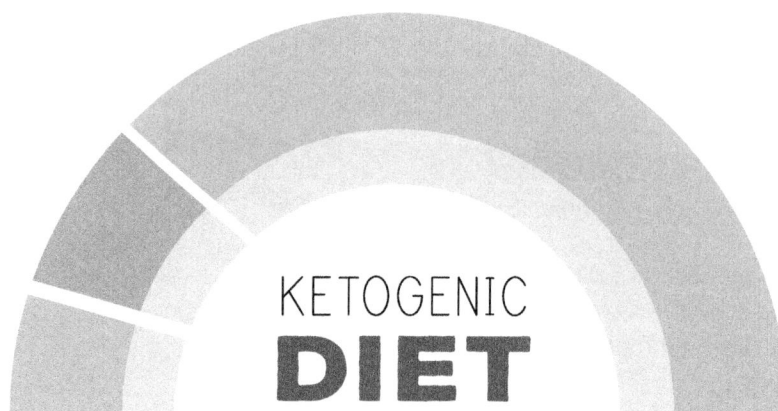

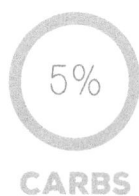

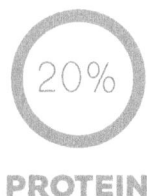

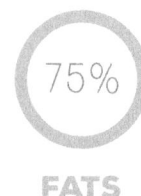

KETOGENIC
DIET

5%
CARBS

20%
PROTEIN

75%
FATS

CHAPTER 4

Foods to Avoid

Every diet plan has two major parts to it: things you can eat and things you cannot eat. We have spoken at length about the things you can eat, why they are important and how they help. Now it's time to look on the flip side - things not to eat and why you should not be eating them.

PROCESSED FOODS

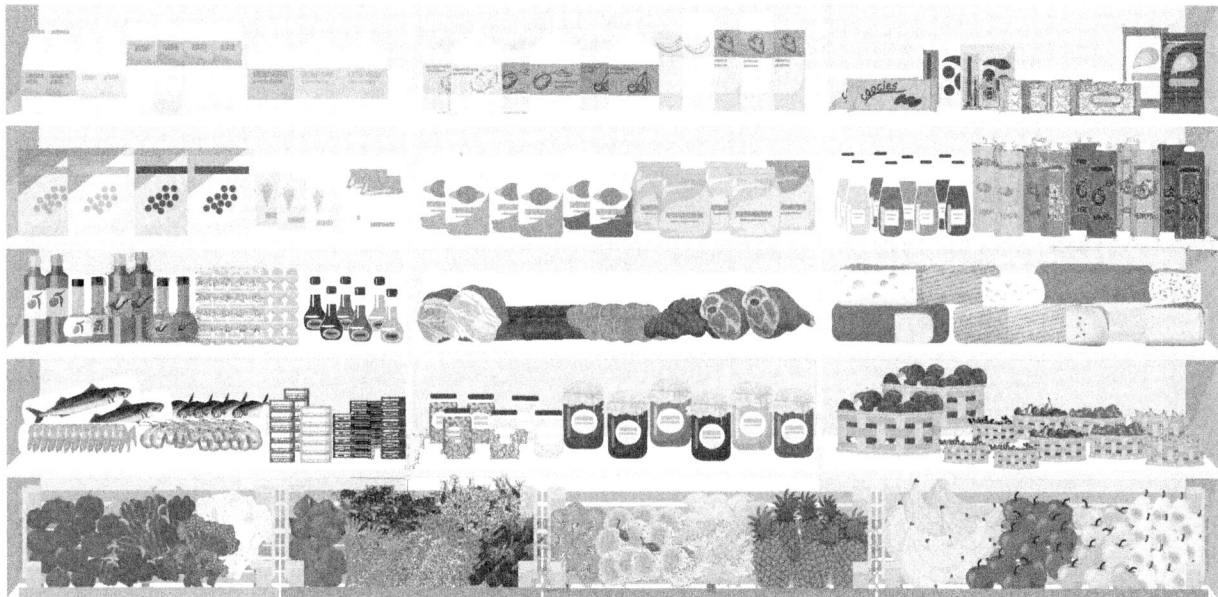

The top of this list is any type of processed food. They are carbohydrate headquarters and should be skipped altogether during your grocery runs.

Mother Nature has all the foods that we require, and the healthiest option is to use it all naturally. Processed foods are filled with preservatives and chemicals. These need to be avoided at all costs.

A good idea is to make a habit of reading the Nutritional Facts labels on foods. A word of caution here, even food labels have an uncanny ability to "hide" important information. Often you can look at a label and see "Sugars 0g", and feel that it's something worth buying. But when you look a couple of lines above that you will see "Total Carbohydrate" which could well be in double digits. A rule of thumb is to not focus on the one-line item when looking at a label. Read the whole thing and then decide.

BOXED CEREALS

Keep your guard up when it comes to boxed cereals. Most popular brands are pretty much devoid of anything which can nourish your body. The box will say a lot of fancy things on it, but one look at the label and you will know that it's something to stay away from. Unless you can find something that is natural with a high amount of fiber and low or no carbs in it, it is best to stay away.

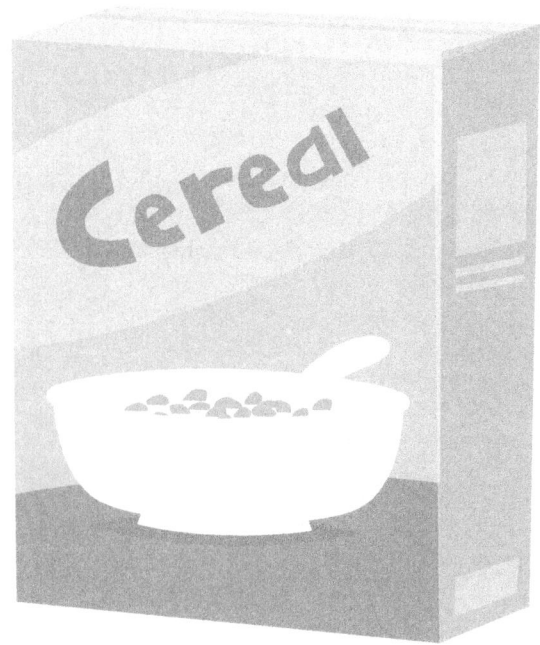

WHITE FLOURS & WHITE RICE

White bread, pasta, and white rice have been stripped of the majority of nutrients and are full of starch. And starches are pure carbohydrates. You can guess what starch leads to: a glucose filled trip which will affect every possible body part in a negative way. So stay away from white bread and its comrades.

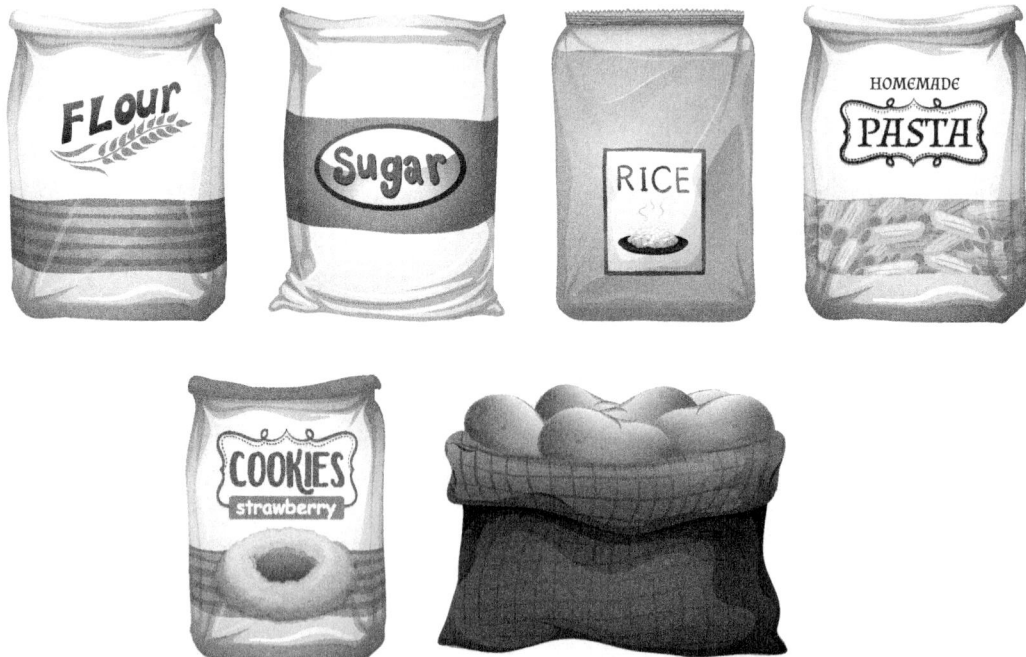

LEGUMES

Legumes, which include beans, lentils, peas and peanuts, seem like they would be an ally because they are so full of protein. Unfortunately, they are also full of carbs. For example, 100 grams of kidney beans contains 24 grams of protein but they also contain 35 grams of the carbs you should avoid. Since legumes do provide a lot of protein, it may be a good idea to keep your daily consumption in the 20-50 gram count. (see "Counting Carbs" below).

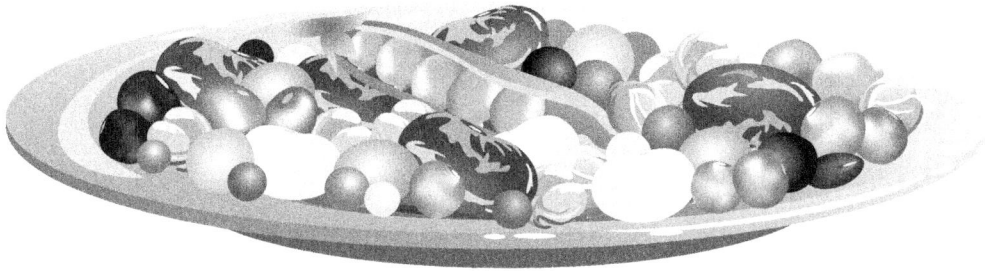

ALCOHOL

Alcohol is a tricky one. Beer should not be on your drinking list as just one beer will take up a large chunk of your carb limit for the day. Pure alcohols, such as whiskey, vodka, brandy, gin and tequila has no fats or carbs. When you drink alcohol, the first organ that gets affected negatively is your liver. When your liver tries to break down alcohol, it damages its cells. You need to protect your liver, especially in a Ketogenic Diet because this is where all your precious ketones are made.

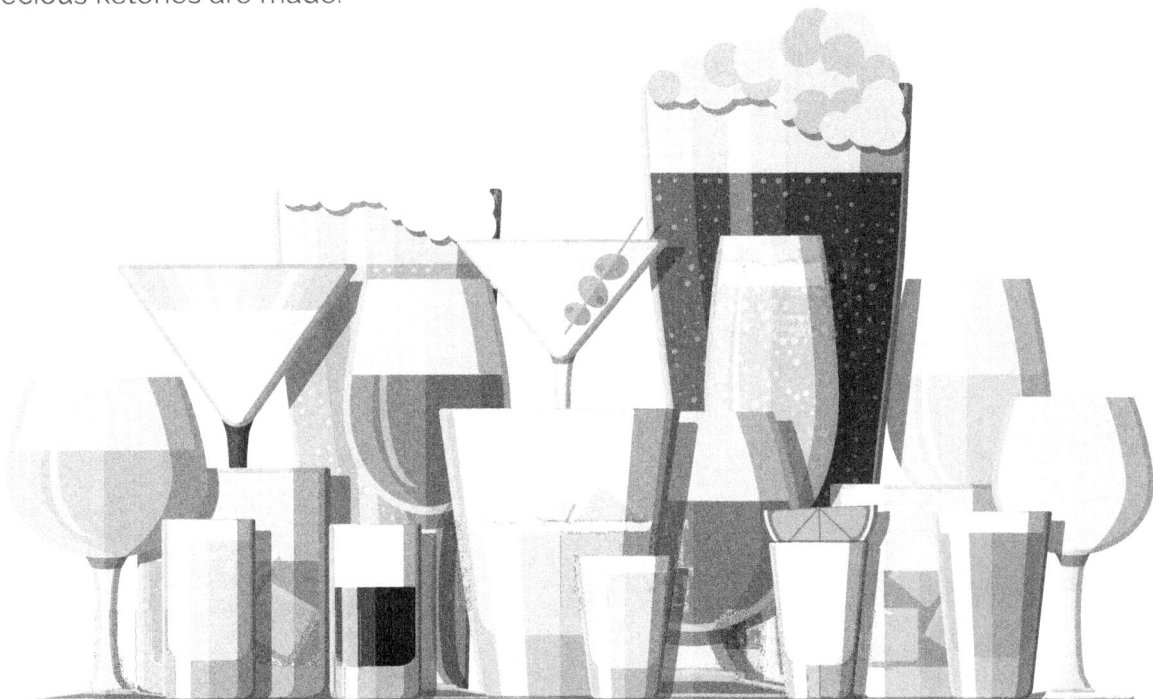

COUNTING CARBS

An important factor to understand is knowing how to choose the carbs that are OK and which you should avoid. What you want to consider when determining the quantity of carbs is to pay most attention to "net carbs". To determine the net carbs of most any food, look at the Nutritional Facts table on the foods you buy.

Use this formula:

Total Carbohydrate minus Dietary Fiber equals Net Carbs. For example, in a typical avocado, there are a total of twelve grams of carbohydrates. However, subtract the ten grams of dietary fiber and the net carbs is only two. This is less than 1.5% of the whole avocado. On the other hand, a typical apple has 25 grams of total carbohydrates of which only 4 are dietary fiber. Net carbs of an apple are 20 grams which is 21% of the whole apple. A huge difference!

Apple Nutrition Facts

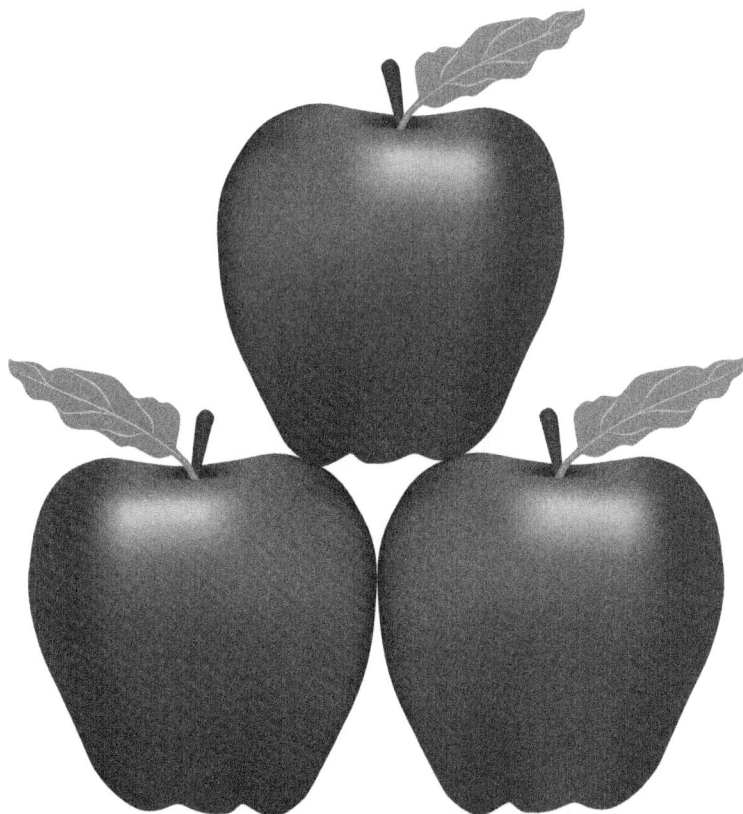

Nutrition Facts

Serving Size 1 Apple (medium)	132 g

Amount Per Serving	
Calories 95	Calories from fat 3

	% Daily Value*
Total Fat 0g	0%
Saturated Fat 0g	0%
Trans Fat 0g	
Cholesterol 0g	0%
Sodium 2mg	0%
Total Carbohydrate 25g	8%
Dietary Fiber 4g	17%
Sugars 19g	
Protein 0g	
Vitamin A	2%
Vitamin C	14%
Calcium	1%
Iron	1%

*Percent Daily Values are based on a 2,000 calorie diet. Your daily values may be higher or lower depending on your calorie needs.

CHAPTER 5

The Keto Diet for Rapid Weight Loss

If you tell anyone that you are working towards weight loss, their response often is something like: "You need to go on a low-carb diet." But you need to understand, it's not that simple and there are many significant differences between a Keto Diet and a low-carb diet.

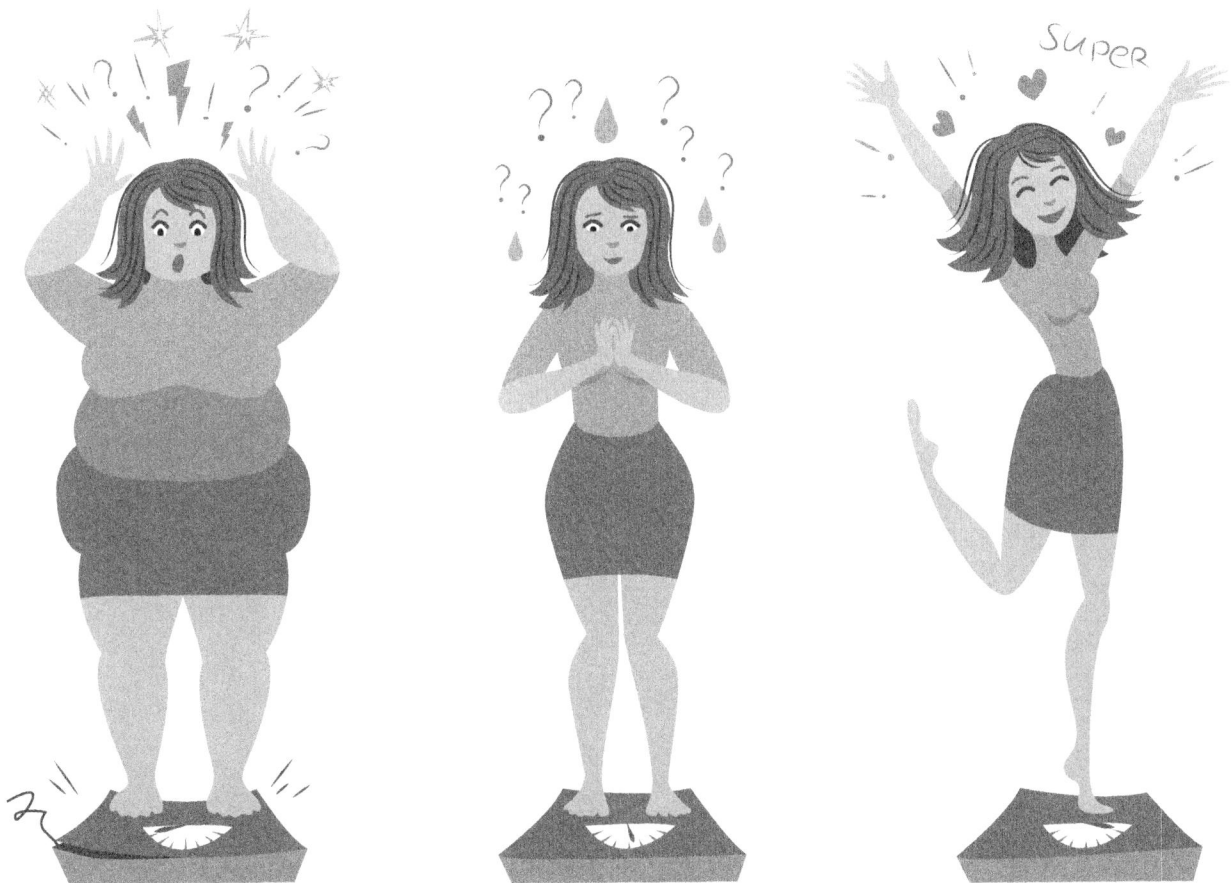

Keto vs Low-carb

If you ask anyone what the definition is of 'low' as in a low-carb diet, you may not get an exact answer. A lot of times, counting carbs can lead to seemingly random choices when looking only at the carb content of a food and deciding whether it should be on your diet or not.

Since there is no defined limit, you may still be eating a lot of carbs and not know it. If you take away carbs from your body and do not replenish it with an alternative source, it will not make you healthy. It will make you hungry, which in turn will make you eat more. On the other hand, Keto has defined limits associated with it and it provides an alternate fuel for your body by using fats.

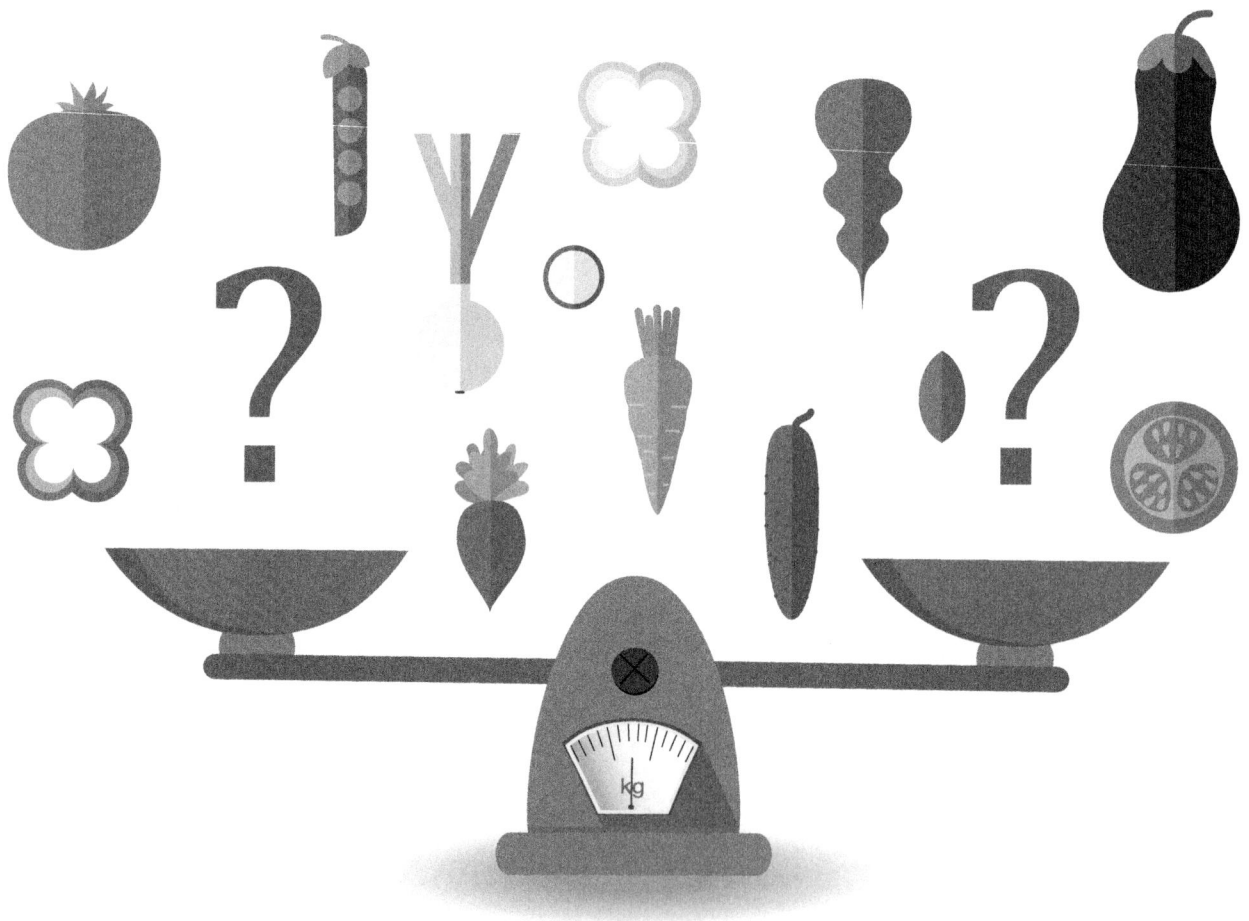

Keto vs Paleo

Many many thousands of years ago when people lived in caves, the diet used to be anything that could be gathered or hunted. The Paleo Diet is designed to shift people back onto the same diet. The Paleo Diet focuses on lean meats, fish, fruits, vegetables, nuts, and seeds. The core idea behind Paleo is that the human body is not meant for the modern diet. According to the theory, the new changes in diet brought about by the advent of farming have outpaced your body's ability to adapt.

However, the drawback with Paleo is that there is generally no controlling or manipulating of carbs, proteins, and fats. Therefore, it is at the opposite end of the spectrum when compared to the Keto Diet. Keto is supposed to not only help with weight loss but it is also supposed to be a "healing diet" where it heals the cells and your body .

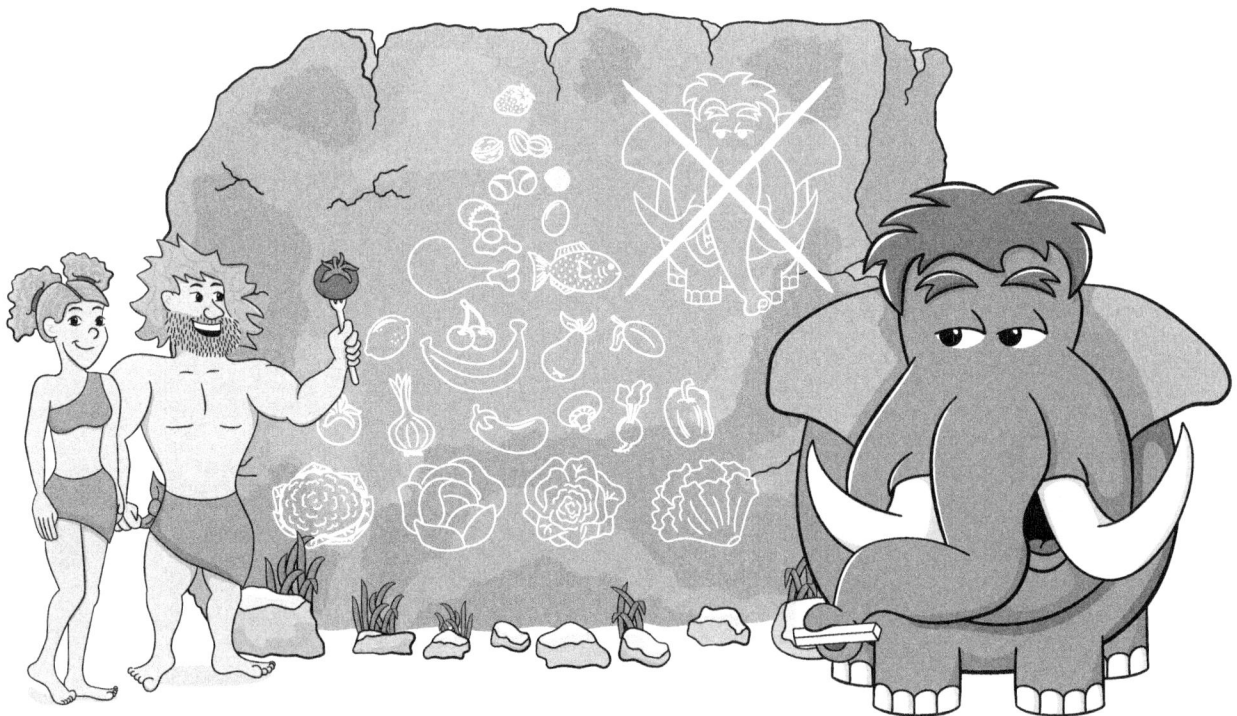

Keto vs Atkins

There are certainly similarities between the Atkins Diet and the Keto Diet. Both are low-carb, high fat diets. But with Atkins, you consume low-carb meals only temporarily whereas in Keto, you continue the diet without changing its basic structure in order to maintain your ideal health and weight. By survey, people often have fewer cravings and eat less calories on the Keto Diet.

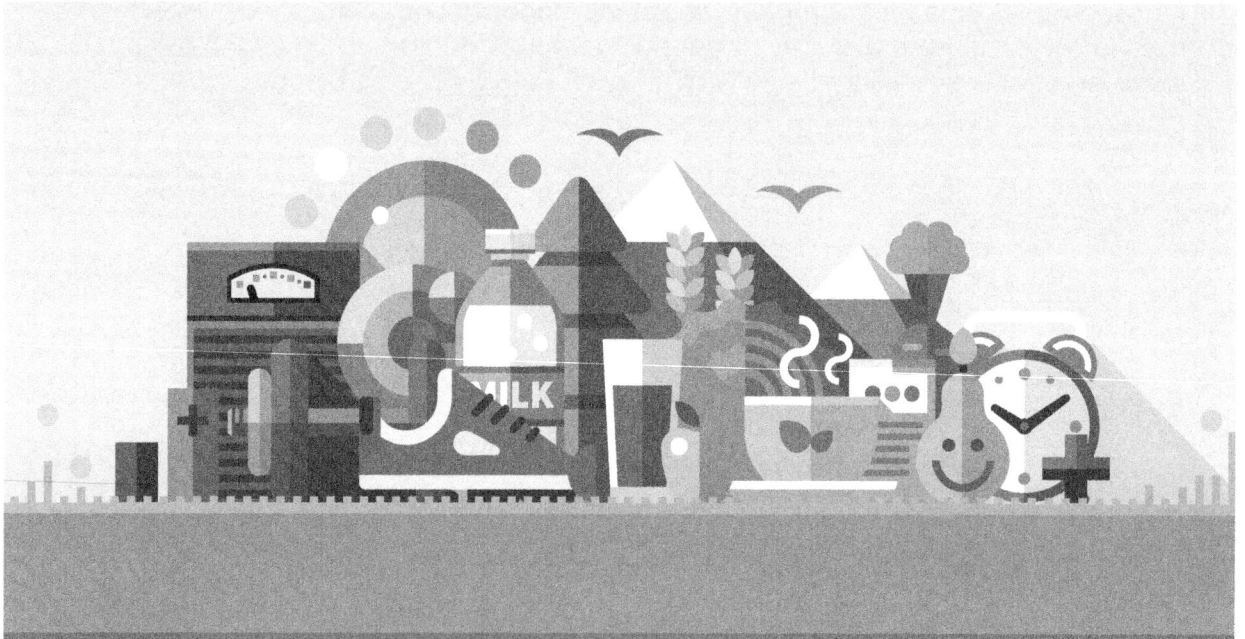

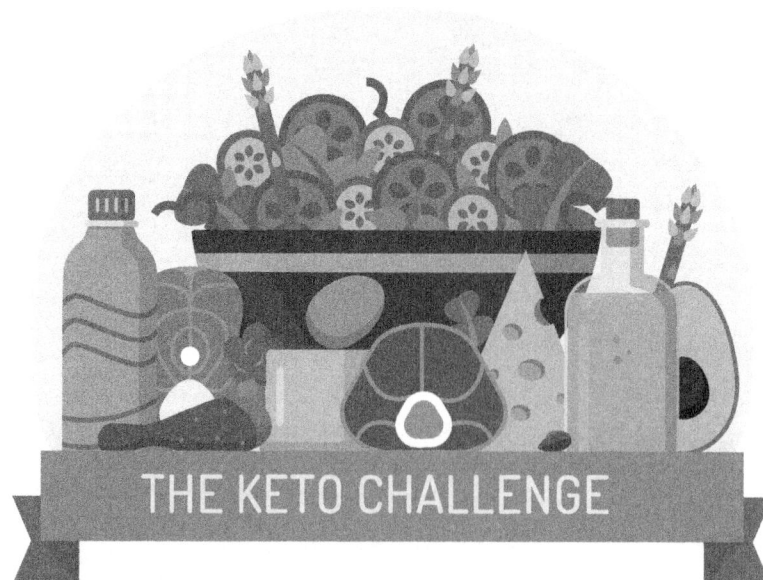

THE KETO CHALLENGE

The Ketogenic Diet

Low-carbs are only one aspect of the Keto Diet. It not only leads you on your way to losing weight, but it also takes your body to an enhanced state of health and well-being. You feel stronger and more energized, which means no unhealthy snacks can sneak up on you when you have hunger pangs. You control your eating, but you are eating better and healthier.

It's for these reasons that so many people around the world are embracing this amazing diet. Its scientific underpinnings ensure that it works. Ketogenic is not a term coined by some new-age guru, it is a scientifically proven process with nearly a hundred years of history that has been validated and tested by many studies and researches.
Ketosis is a state when, in the absence of carbohydrates, your body is compelled to use the alternative source of energy and it burns the fats stored in your body for this purpose. That is why the Keto Diet has been so successful. This is not something new, it has been around for ages.

The ancient Indian physicians used to fast for days, which led to ketosis which they saw enriched their minds and bodies. Since the early 1920s, the Keto Diet was used to treat and help epileptic children. The Keto Diet is a process which, like any other process, is difficult in the beginning because you are trying to break habits which have been formed over the years. But once you go through the process, you see a healthier and stronger you. Another feature that makes Keto stand out is that there is no deprivation or hunger involved. You do not stop eating, you choose to eat in a better and healthier way.

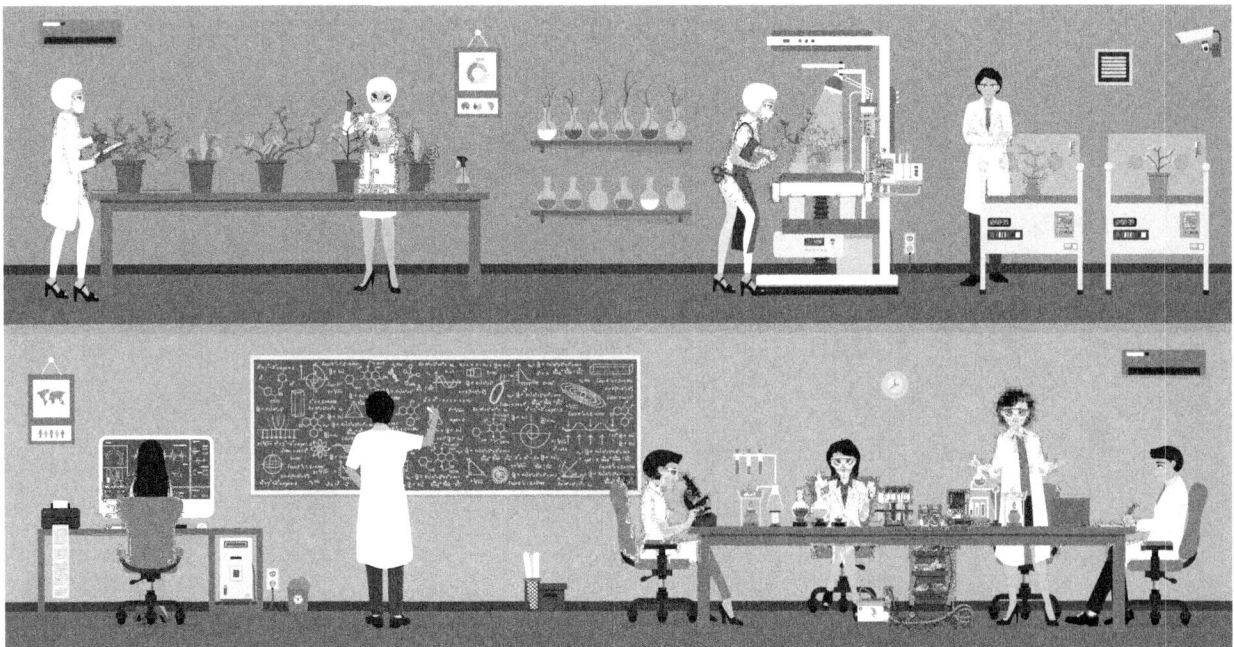

Ketosis Explained

Ketosis is not a spell conjured by Harry Potter. It's a natural occurrence where your body looks for a different pathway to an energy source when it's deprived of its usual path.

At some point in our lives, we have all experienced ketosis, maybe after a strenuous exercise session or when mom forgot to leave lunch in the fridge and we are too lazy to make anything ourselves and therefore your body has started producing ketones to keep us working. Unfortunately, many people eat too much sugar and carbs which prevents ketosis from happening.

A pack of cigarettes has all the warnings on it, yet a smoker ignores all of them. Similarly, we all know the negative effects of excessive sugar and carbs in our bodies, yet we devour them daily. And as a result, we face health issues not limited to weight gain such as diabetes, fatigue, acne, heart disease and so on.

The more you control your intake of carbs, the more your body can produce ketones. Under normal circumstances, fats are stored as an emergency reserve by your body, but during ketosis, it becomes the main source of fuel and you can control it by what you eat and how you eat it.

The Ketogenic Diet is not just a process you follow for a few days and then revert to a diet full of carbs. It is a lifestyle because, as we have mentioned before, so many times it has benefits that go beyond a few pounds off your belly.

Before starting a Keto Diet, you need to first create your goals. Do you simply want to lose weight or are you concerned about your overall health? Is a disease showing its early signs? Always remember, a Keto Diet can be adjusted to suit your needs and goals.

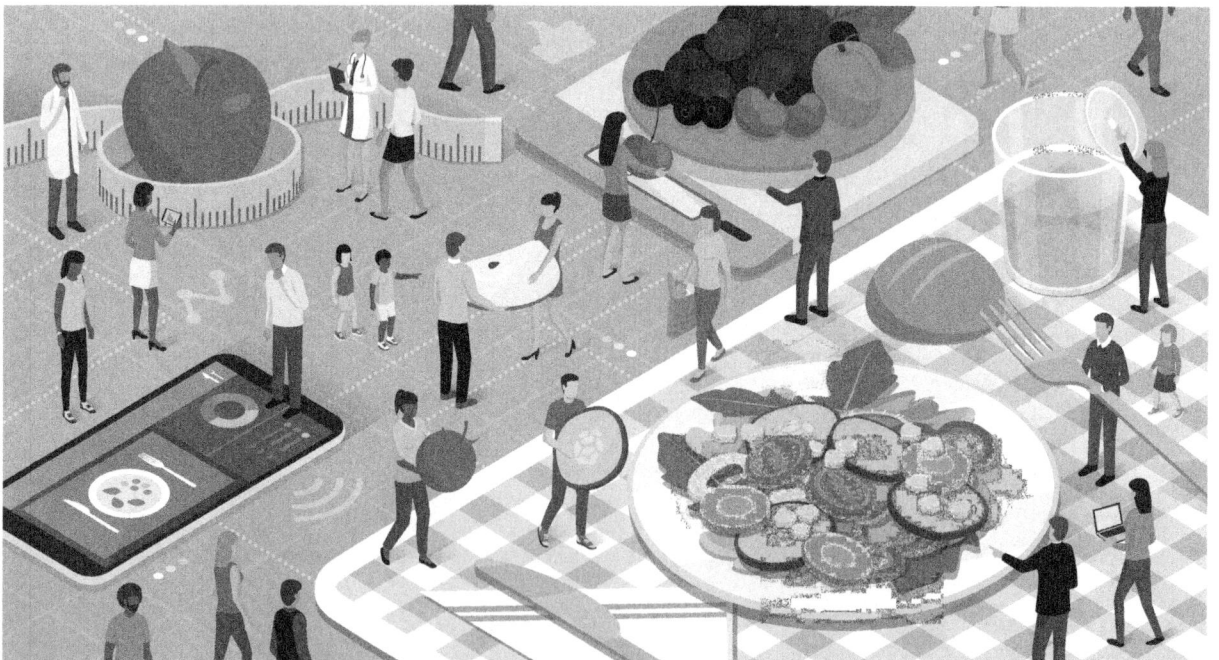

Keto Symptoms

The body may need a bit of time to adapt to using fat as its main energy source, especially if your body has been running on carbohydrates as its main energy source for a long period of time. Sometimes there are some symptoms involved during this period of adaptation. These symptoms are called the "keto flu," an experienced set of side-effects associated with carbohydrate withdrawal. Some of these symptoms include: headaches, dizziness, cramps/sore muscles, nausea, fatigue, irritability, mood swings, cravings, stomach pain/constipation, brain fog and insomnia. The "keto flu" symptoms usually disappear by themselves within a few days, as the body adapts. Here are a few tips to help you cure some of these symptoms faster if you experience the 'keto flu' symptoms. Drink a glass of water with a teaspoon of sea salt stirred into it at least once a day. You can also have bone broth as a tasty alternative with salt. In addition having electrolytes and B vitamins can help with this transition period. Make sure you also drink water when you are thirsty. Another tip is in the beginning stages take it easy with exercise and increase the intensity over a few weeks. Once you are over the "keto flu" symptoms you will soon be reaping all the benefits of your body being in a state of ketosis.

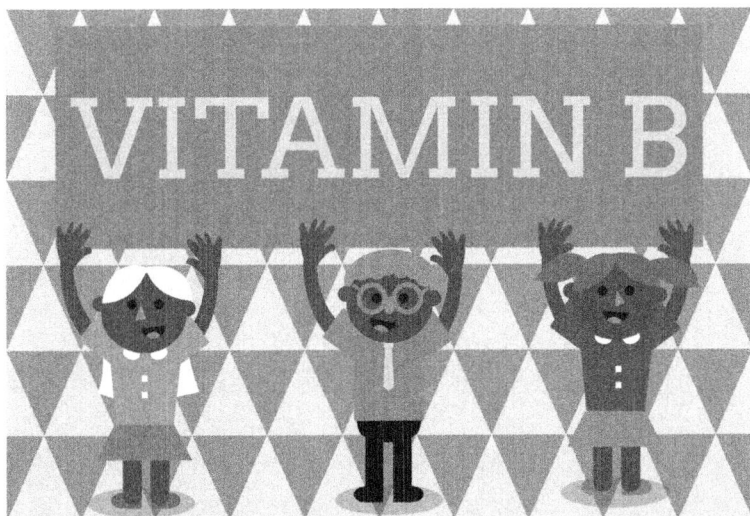

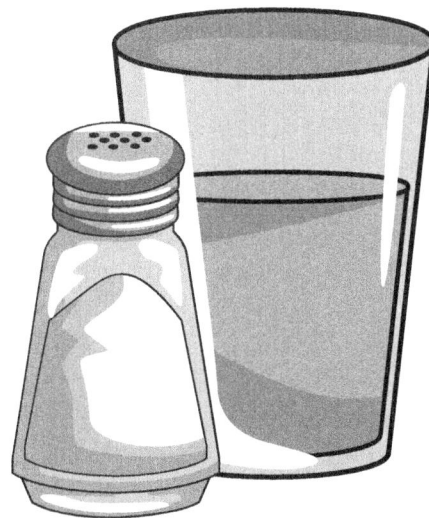

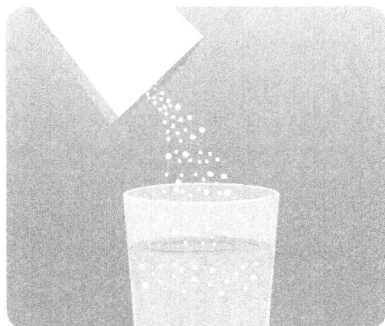

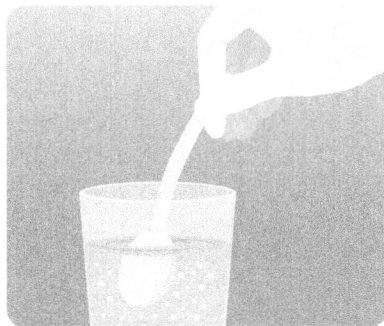

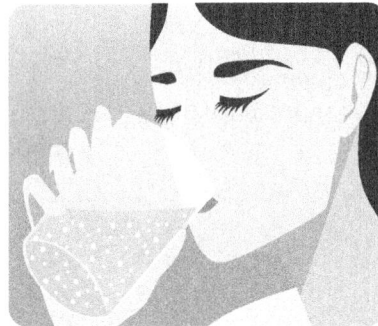

Intermittent Fasting on a Keto Diet

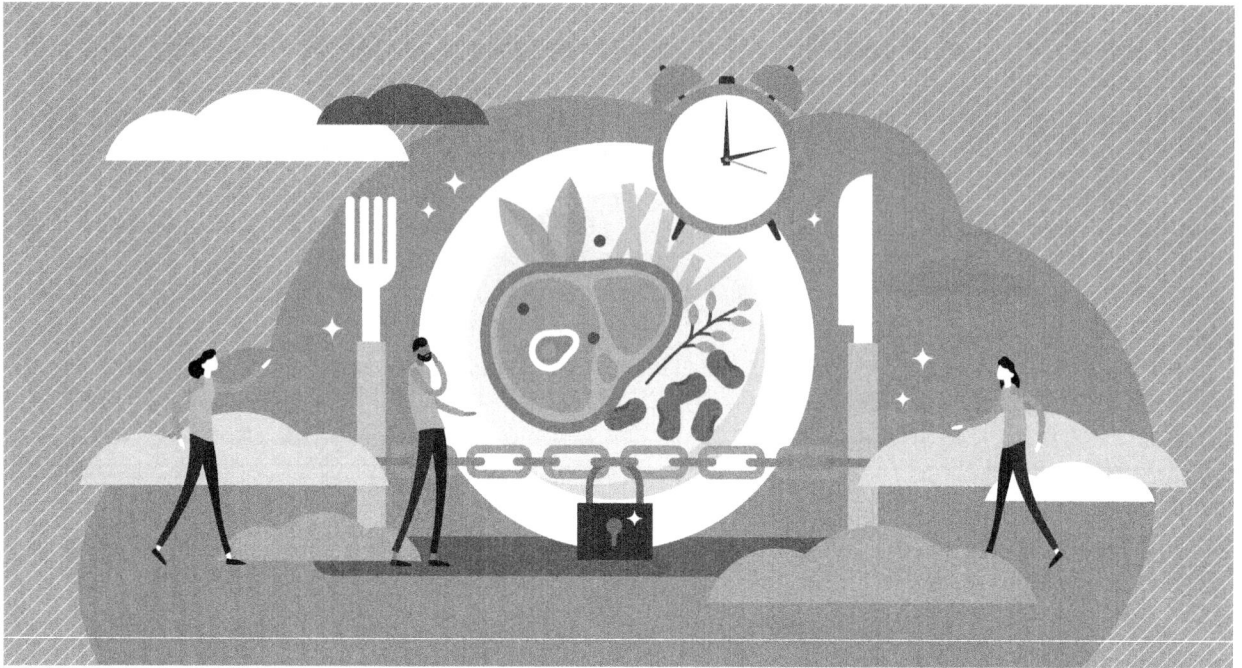

Intermittent fasting is a critically important step one can take for accelerated weight loss and maintaining ketosis.

One can take the Keto Diet to the next level by implementing a scheduled eating pattern called intermittent fasting. The benefit of intermittent fasting is that it shifts the body more readily into ketosis and one will discover that going longer periods of time without eating will be no problem since the body will be feeding off stored fat. Though one may be on the keto diet primarily to return to an ideal weight, the greatest benefit of intermittent fasting is the increase in health and resistance to diseases. Many studies show that this type of fasting while on the Keto Diet, helps the body's ability to ward off diseases such as cancer, Alzheimer's, Diabetes and more will be strengthened as a result.

Here's how this works: One already goes on an intermittent fast, every night. One is asleep for seven hours or so during which time one eats no food, right? That is many hours of fasting already. One can take it up a notch. Instead of eating three meals per day, possibly even with snacking in between, one would first start by cutting out any snacks between meals. Then start skipping breakfast to extend the fasting period. This can be done on a gradient by slowly having breakfast later and later in the day until you are eating "breakfast" at lunchtime. The goal for intermittent fasting would be to only eat two meals per day within a six-hour window. One meal around lunchtime and the last one at dinner time. That would give one a daily fasting period of up to eighteen hours. One cup of coffee or tea first thing in the morning is fine if needed.

One will soon discover that eating on this schedule is very simple. One will feel energetic, mentally sharp and surprisingly one won't even feel hungry during these fasting periods. Many people are also amazed at the weight loss boost one gets from intermittent fasting.

CHAPTER 6

Let the Keto Journey Begin

You have finally decided. Take the leap into a healthier, more fit and with knowing that science has proven the workability of your decision. Your journey will lead you on a path of not only better health, but also towards a strong mental state. So, let's get the ball rolling and make it happen!

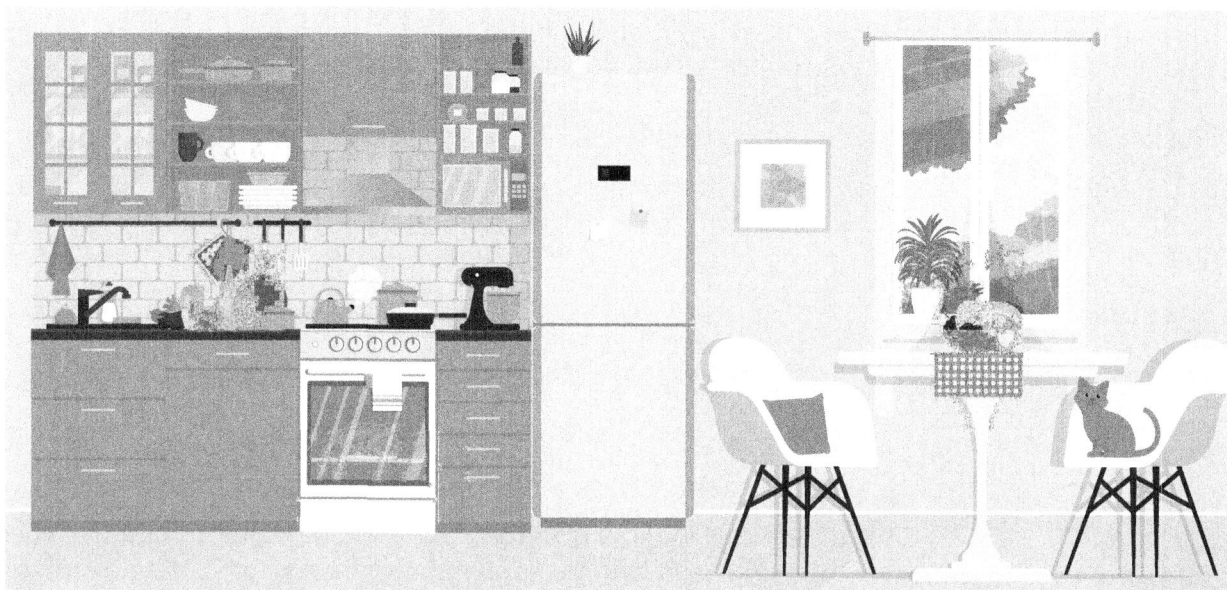

Time to Clean Out the Pantry

That pantry in your kitchen has had years of being restocked with sugars and carbs. It needs a major spring cleaning. Take all these items and put them in a box to donate or discard. Involve your family, it helps if you all are in it together. If they don't want to, it's okay. Your results will show them the way.

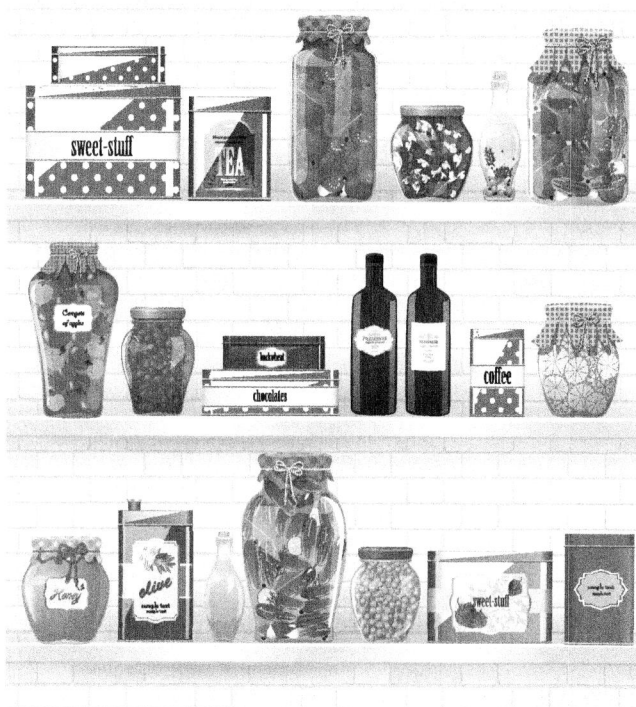

Weigh Yourself

You need to know where you are so you can measure how far you have come. You may notice a little gain initially, but don't lose hope.

Remember it's a process and it will get better as your body gets used to it. You don't have to weigh yourself every day and stress over when the scale doesn't go in the right direction. Losing weight on the Keto Diet is not always linear. It can happen in fits and starts. Just hang in there and soon enough you will enjoy the results.

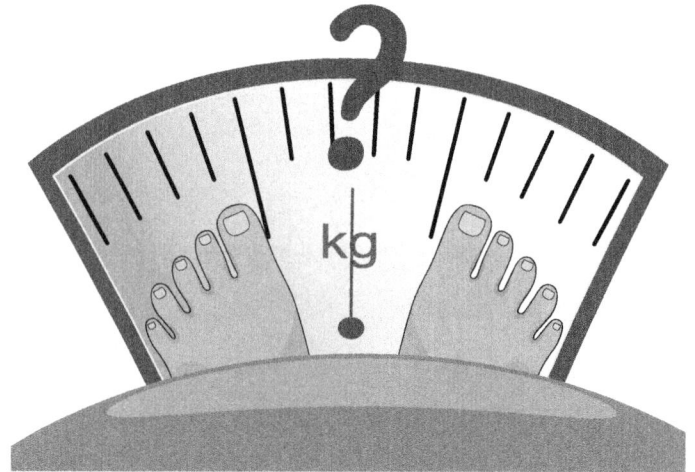

Get Smart with Substitutes

Remember those cheesecakes that you loved so much? Or those mashed potatoes which were on your plate every time? Yes, you won't be eating them on a Keto Diet, but you will be able to find low-carb substitutes.

There are always recipes that will provide you with a similar dish without the negative side effects. Try to swap a carb-rich ingredient of your favorite food with something more keto-friendly. A lettuce wrap is an excellent substitute for a carb-laden taco shell. Grated cauliflower may be the answer to your mashed potato cravings. Ever try the 'courgetti'? It's courgette spaghetti. We are all born creative, let's use a bit of it when looking at the things we eat.

We at Ketoveo have published a number of cookbooks containing literally thousands of recipes in order to to make it easy for you to choose and make healthy, tasty and fulfiling keto-friendly breakfasts, lunches, dinners and desserts. Go to Ketoveo.com to see all of our various cookbook choices.

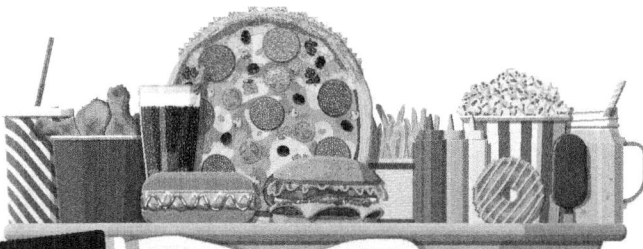

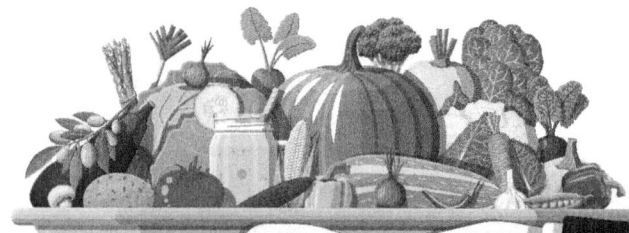

Condiments are not Your Friend

If you ever thought that ketchup is healthy, think again. Ketchup is filled with sugar. Read the label of your everyday condiments and you will be surprised at what you find. Keep your guard up against salad dressings at restaurants. It's better to ask what they are made of instead of eating and going on a sugar trip.

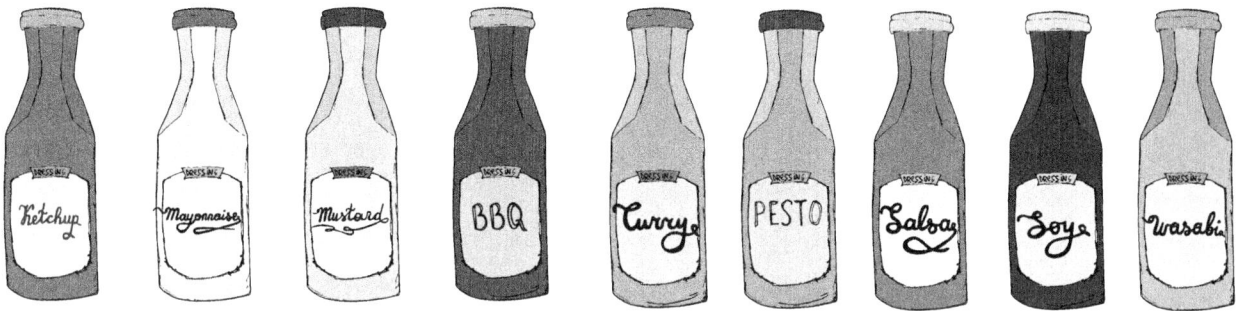

Watch Your Ketones

Keep an eye on your ketone levels. It is an important step to know what is happening inside of your liver with those ketones. It is a simple urine test. Do it first thing in the morning to get the most accurate reading.

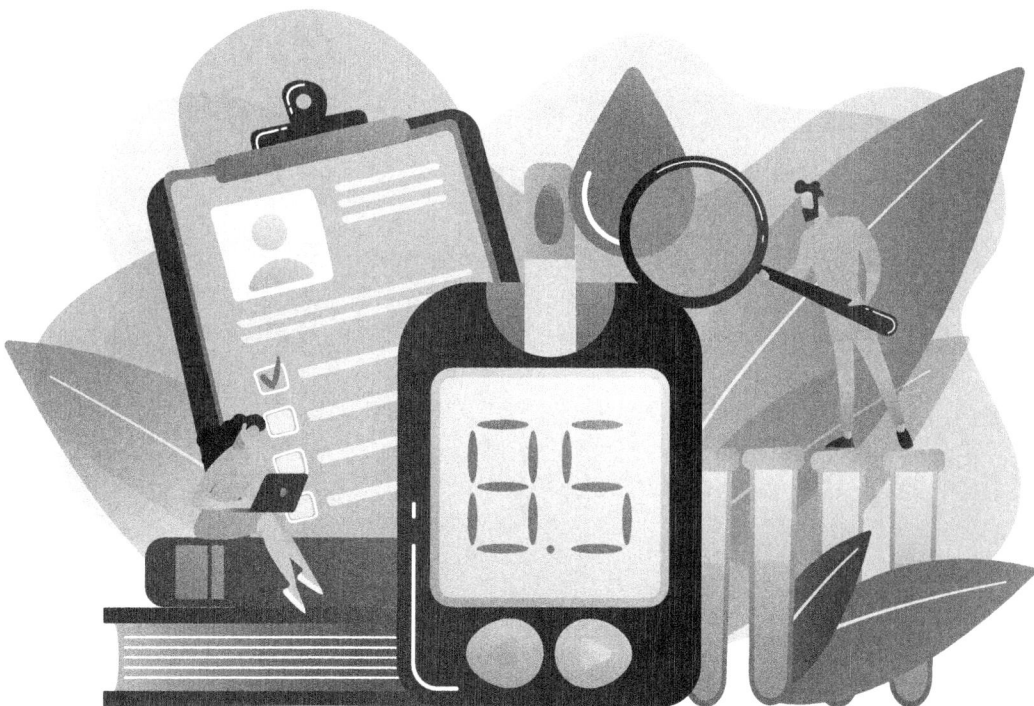

What About Eating Out?

You might be thinking: A Keto Diet would mean an end to eating out, right? Absolutely not! You merely have to choose your foods wisely, always keeping in mind what your goals are in terms of carbs, proteins, and fats. There are plenty of things available on most good restaurant menus to choose from so you need not worry overmuch. This will keep you on track and allow you to still enjoy your favorite restaurants.

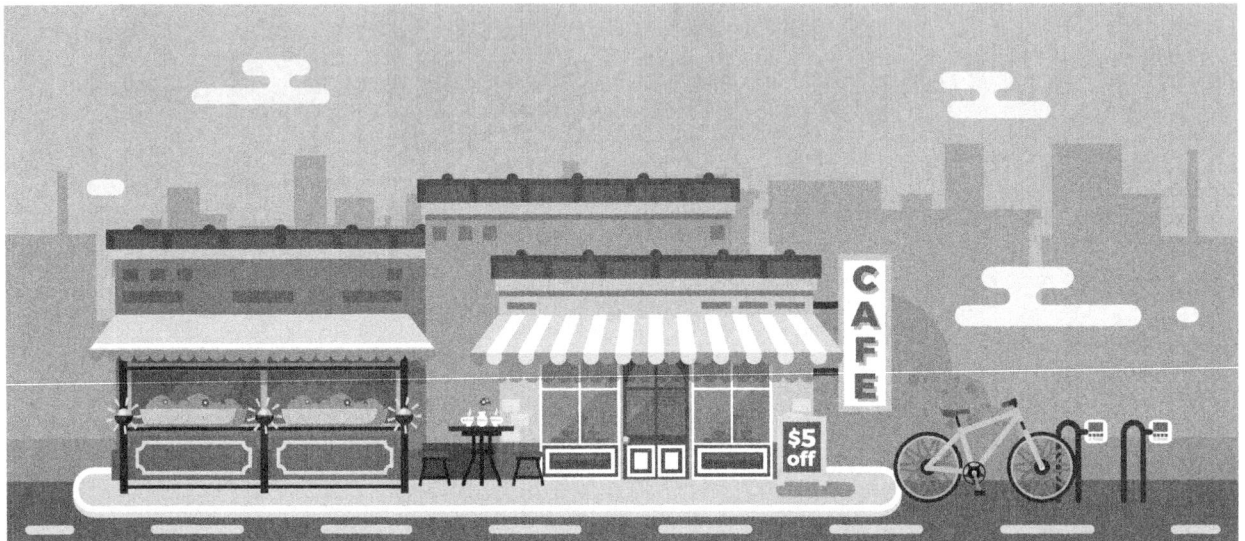

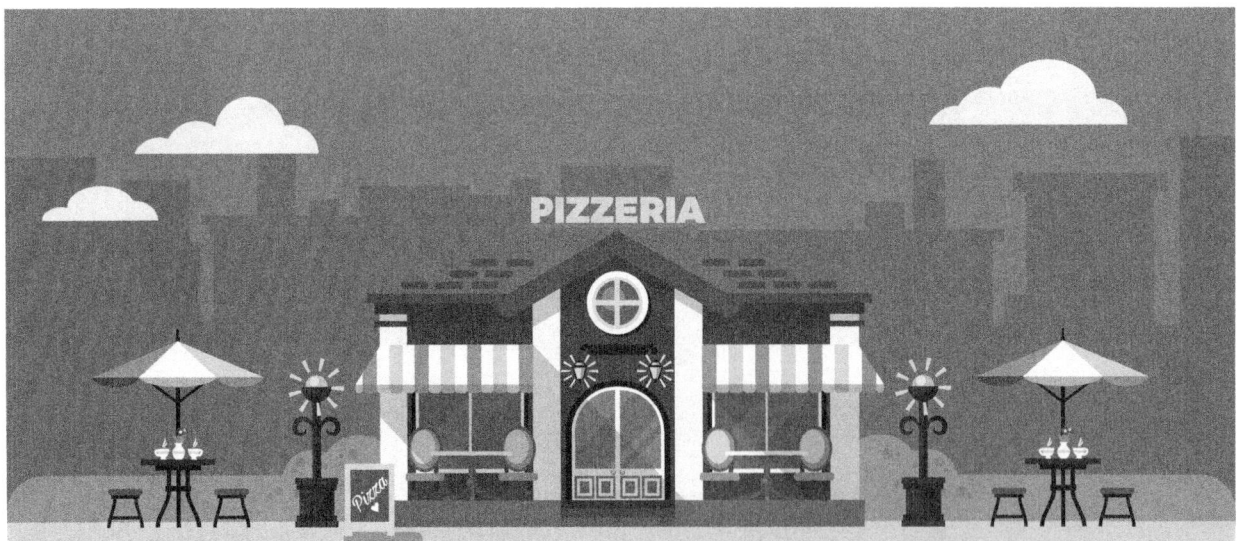

Get Your Protein & Exercise

A Keto Diet with plenty of protein will help your body build muscle as long as you include a healthy amount of exercise. Make exercise a part of your routine. Keep it simple. If you can't make it to the gym, get creative at home.

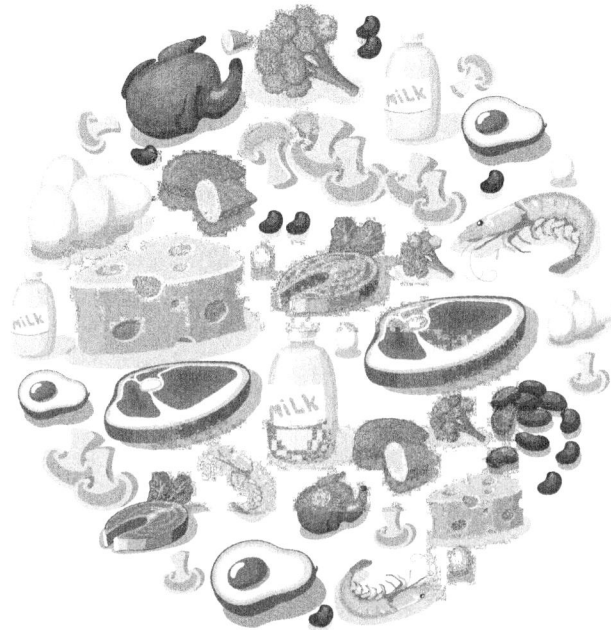

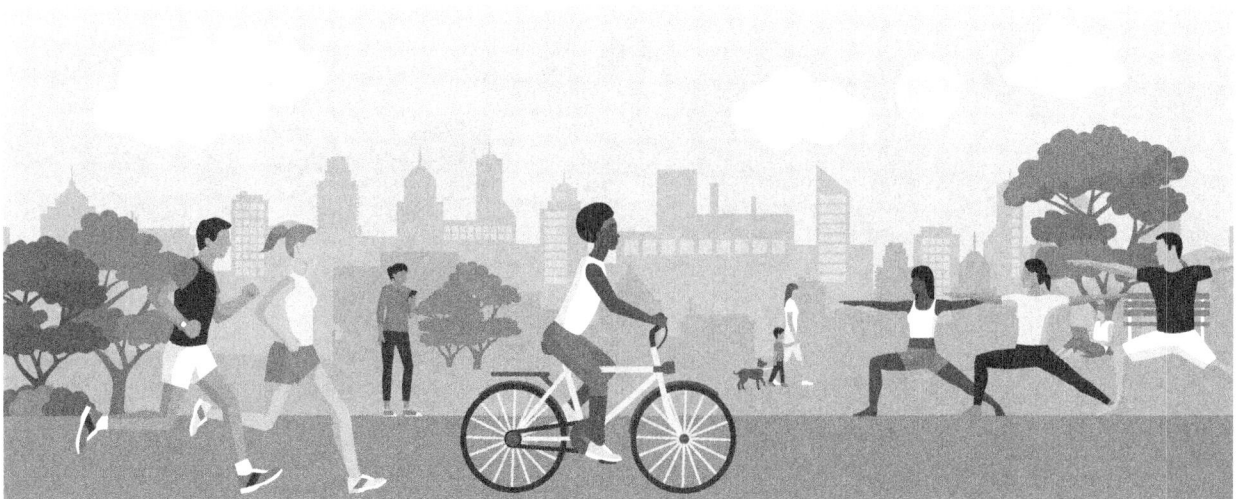

Endgame

In a few months, after having embraced the Keto lifestyle, you will look better, feel better, and you will be amazed at your surge in energy. You have made choices which have tested your willpower, but you have done it.

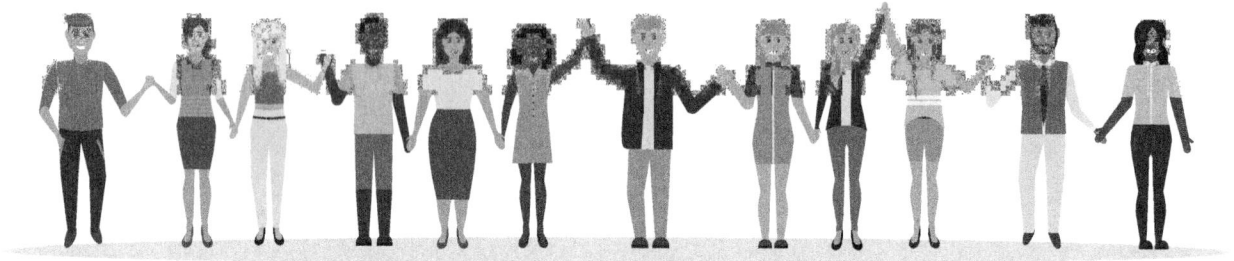

So what is next? Once you have lost those extra pounds or improved your health, you need to keep going. It is often said, 'It's easier to reach the top than it is to stay there." Do not stop, keep going, keep those carbs away and let your ketones do their job. It will enrich you and inspire others around you. You have come a long way, enjoy the journey, enjoy the process. Have a great Keto life.

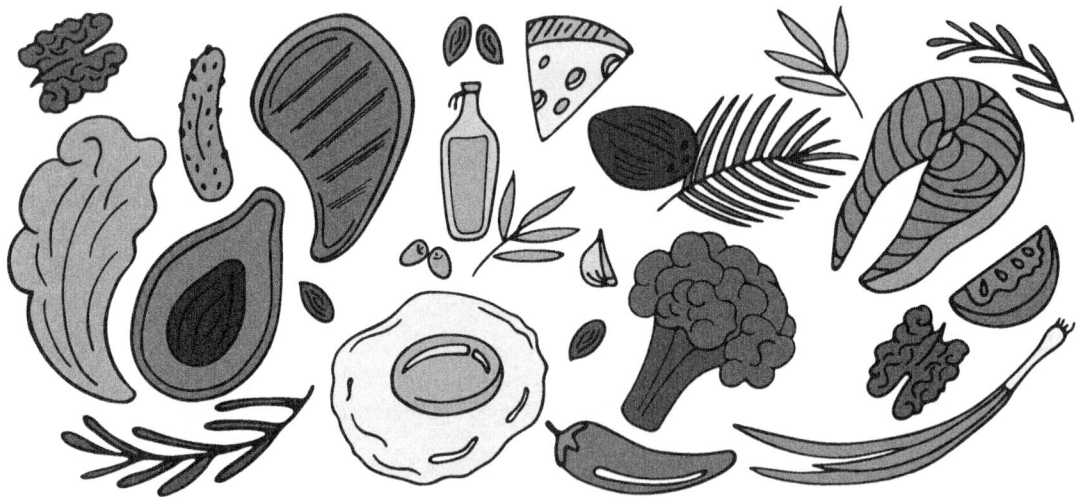

Ketogenic diet

CHAPTER 7

Keto Friendly Food

VEGETABLES PART 1   KETOVEO.COM

0.3g Endive	0.6g Beet greens	0.7g Chicory	0.8g Watercress	1.2g Pak choi (bok choy)
1.4g Kale (cavolo nero)	1.4g Spinach	1.4g Celery	1.4g Collard	1.5g Cucumber
1.5g Samphire	1.5g Mustard greens	1.7g Parsley root (not parsnip!)	1.8g Asparagus	1.8g Radishes
1.8g Mizuna greens	1-2g Lettuce	2.1g Swiss chard	2.1g Zucchini (courgette)	2.1g Arugula (rocket)
2.3g White mushroom	2.6g Napa cabbage	2.6g Potobello mushroom	2.6g Kohlrabi	2.7g Tomatoes
2.9g Green bell pepper	2.9g Eggplant (aubergine)	3g Savoy cabbage	3g Cauliflower	3.2g Green cabbage

BEST ← CARBS → WORST

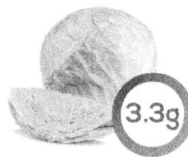 3.3g
White Cabbage

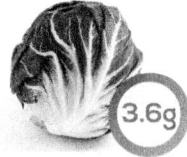 3.6g
Radicchio

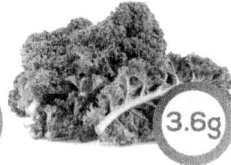 3.6g
Kale (curly)

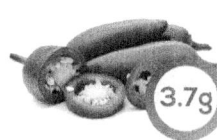 3.7g
Jalapeno peppers

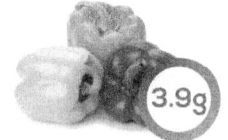 3.9g
Other bell pepper

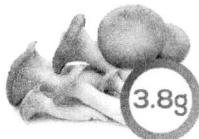 3.8g
Oyster mushroom

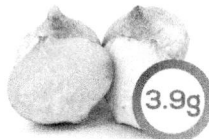 3.9g
Jicama

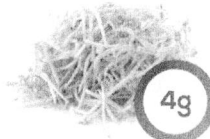 4g
Bean sprouts

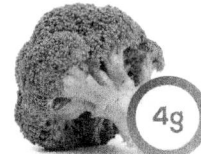 4g
Broccoli

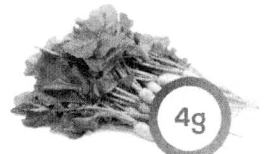 4g
Daikon radish

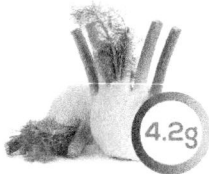 4.2g
Fennel

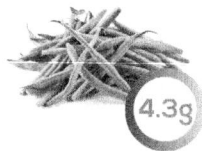 4.3g
Green beans

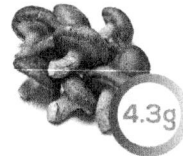 4.3g
Shiitake mushroom

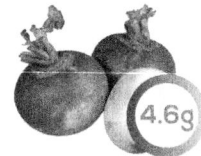 4.6g
Turnip

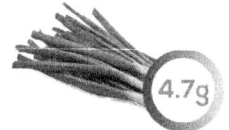 4.7g
Spring Onion

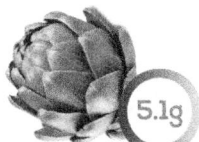 5.1g
Artichoke (globe)

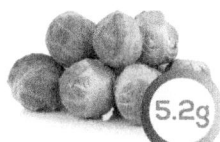 5.2g
Brussel sprouts

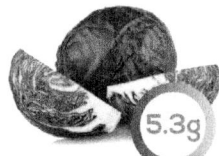 5.3g
Red cabbage

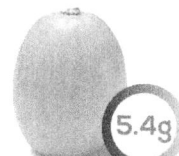 5.4g
Spaghetti squash

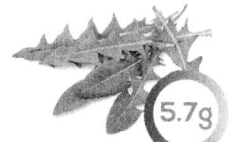 5.7g
Dandelion greens

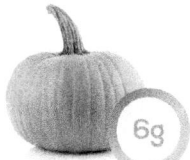 6g
Pie pumpkin

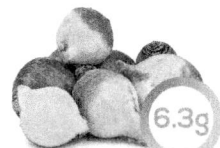 6.3g
Rutabaga (swede)

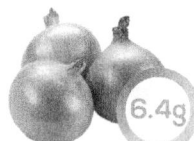 6.4g
Brown onion

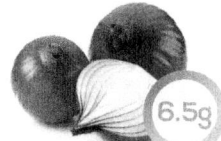 6.5g
Red onion

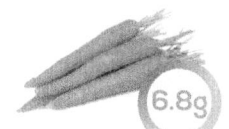 6.8g
Carrot

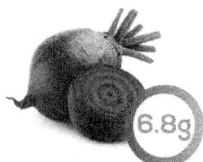 6.8g
Beetroot

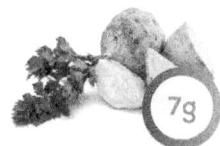 7g
Celeriac

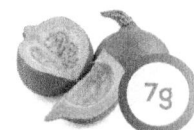 7g
Hokkaido squash

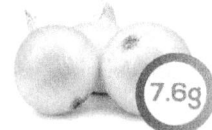 7.6g
White onion

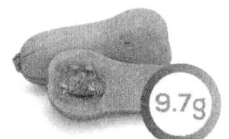 9.7g
Butter squash

BEST　　　　　←　CARBS　→　　　　　**WORST**

40

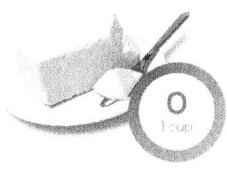

Butter

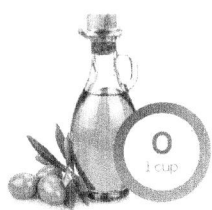

Olive oil

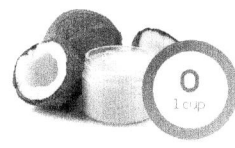

Coconut oil

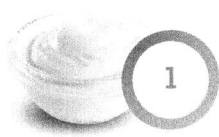

Mayonnaise

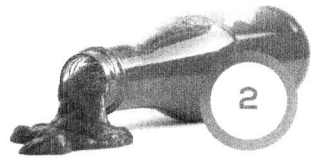

Tabasco / Hot sause

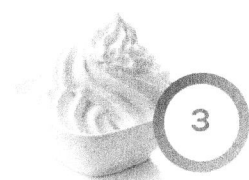

Heavy cream

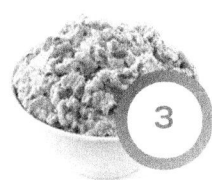

Guacamole

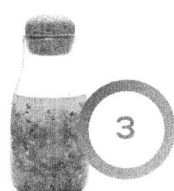

Vinaigrette

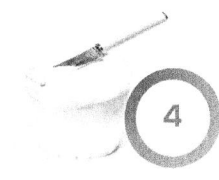

Cream cheese

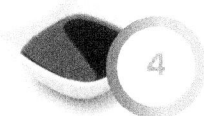

Soy sause

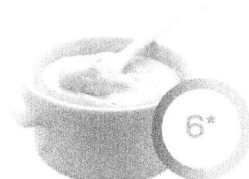

Mustard

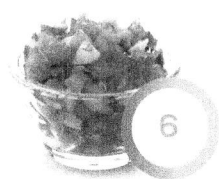

Salsa

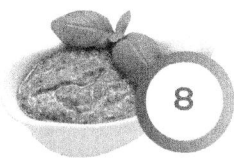

Pesto

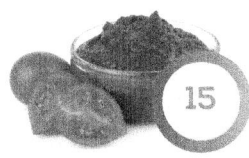

Tomato paste

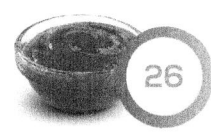

Ketchup

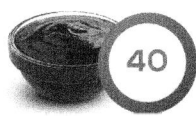

BBQ sause

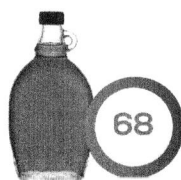

Maple syrup

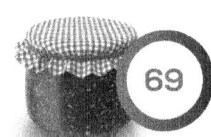

Jam

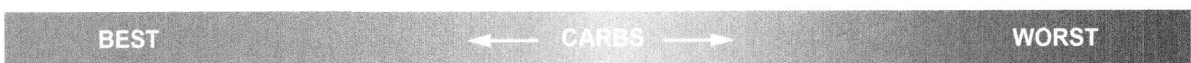

BEST　　　　⟵　CARBS　⟶　　　　WORST

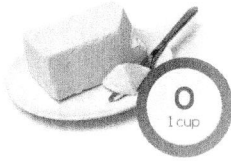
Butter

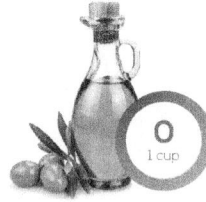
Olive oil

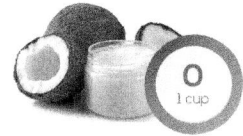
Coconut oil

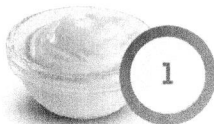
Mayonnaise

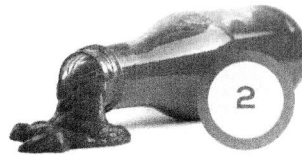
Tabasco / Hot sause

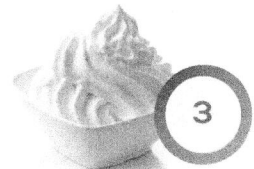
Heavy cream

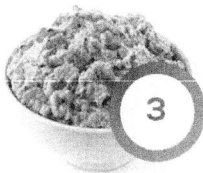
Guacamole

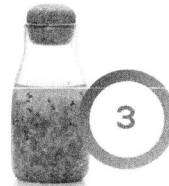
Vinaigrette

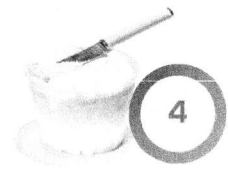
Cream cheese

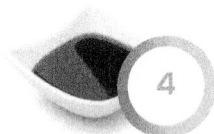
Soy sause

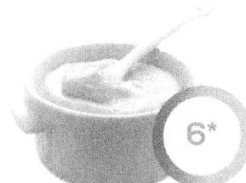
Mustard

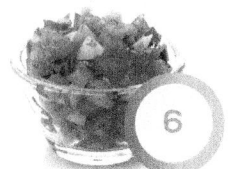
Salsa

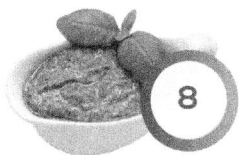
Pesto

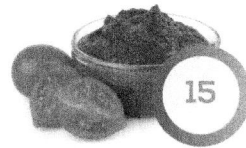
Tomato paste

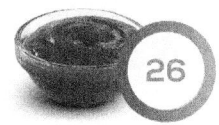
Ketchup

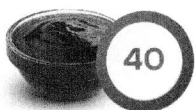
BBQ sause

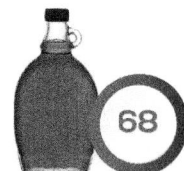
Maple syrup

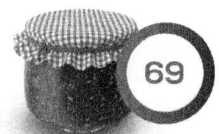
Jam

BEST   ← CARBS →   WORST

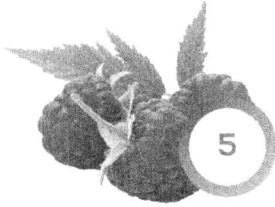
Raspberry — 5

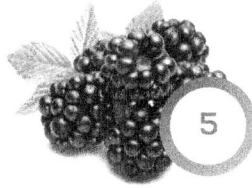
Blackberry — 5

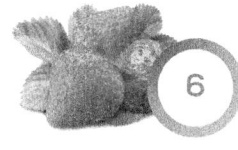
Strawberry — 6

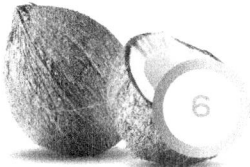
Coconut (Meat) — 6

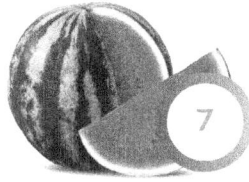
Watermelon — 7

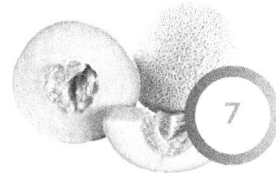
Cantaloupe — 7

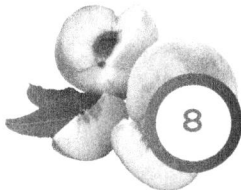
Peach — 8

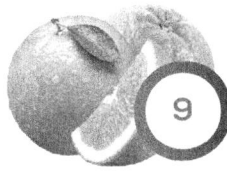
Orange — 9

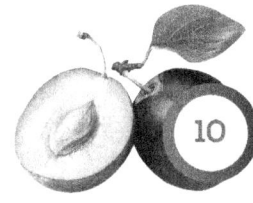
Plum — 10

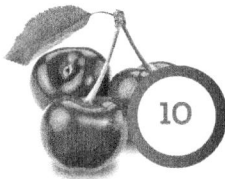
Cherries — 10

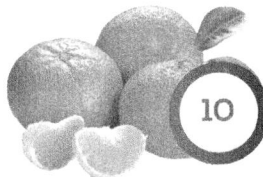
Clementine — 10

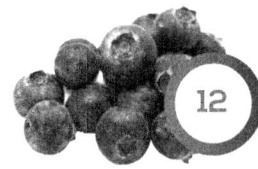
Blueberry — 12

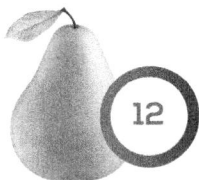
Pear — 12

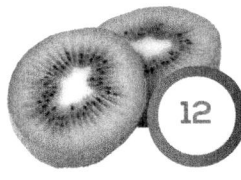
Kiwi — 12

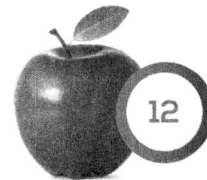
Apple — 12

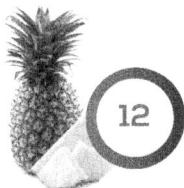
Pineapple — 12

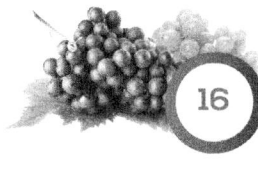
Grapes — 16

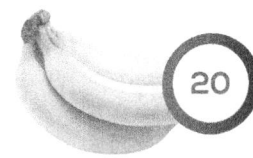
Banana — 20

BEST   ← CARBS →   WORST

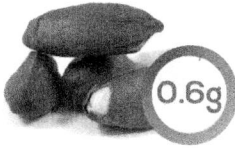 **0.6g**
Pili nuts

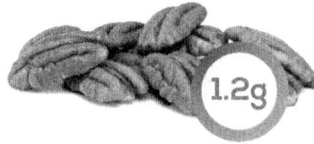 **1.2g**
Pecan

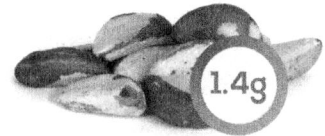 **1.4g**
Brazil nuts

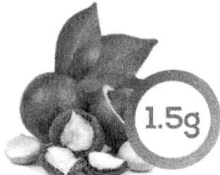 **1.5g**
Macadamia

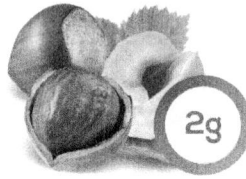 **2g**
Hazelnut

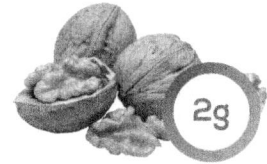 **2g**
Walnut

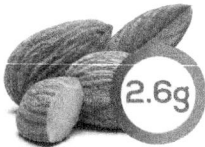 **2.6g**
Almonds

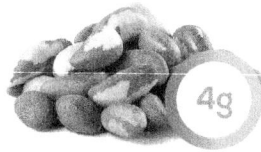 **4g**
Brazil

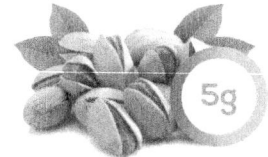 **5g**
Pistachio

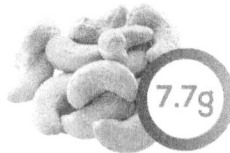 **7.7g**
Cashews

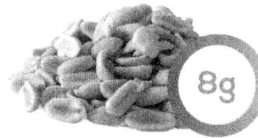 **8g**
Peanut

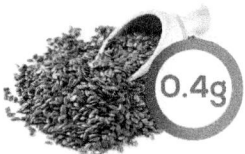 **0.4g**
Flax seeds

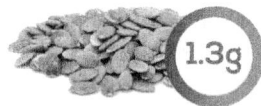 **1.3g**
Pumpkin seeds

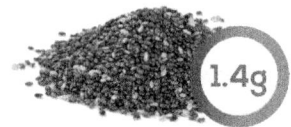 **1.4g**
Chia seeds

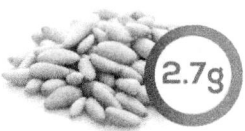 **2.7g**
Pine seeds

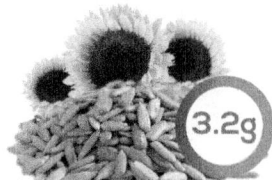 **3.2g**
Sunflower seeds

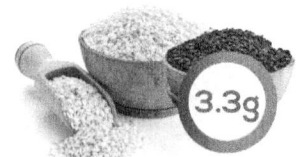 **3.3g**
Sesame seeds

| BEST | ← CARBS → | WORST |

Shopping List

BEEF

- Steak
- Prime Rib
- Veal
- Roast Beef
- Brisket
- Loin
- Ground beef
- Stew meats
- Organs

POULTRY

- Chicken
- Quail
- Turkey
- Organs
- Eggs

PORK

- Bacon
- Ground pork
- Sausage
- Bratwurst
- Pork rinds
- Ham
- Pork chops

SEAFOOD

- Salmon
- Tuna
- Trout
- Cod
- Sardines
- Tilapia
- Shrimp
- Lobster
- Crab
- Bass
- Scallops
- Mussels
- Clams
- Oysters

OTHER
- Deli meats
- Jerky sticks
- Biltong
- Salami
- Goat
- Lamb

LEAFY GREENS

- Spinach
- Kale
- Swiss chard
- Lettuce
- Bok choy
- Watercress
- Endive
- Dandelion greens

CRUCIFEROUS VEGGIES

- Broccoli
- Cauliflower
- Red cabbage
- Green cabbage
- Napa cabbage
- Brussels sprouts

ALL OTHER VEGETABLES AND GREENS

- Avocado
- Asparagus
- Celery
- Spring onion
- Fennel
- Radish
- Kohlrabi
- Jalapeño peppers
- Zucchini
- Eggplant
- Green peppers
- Other bell peppers
- Cucumbers
- Tomatoes
- Spaghetti squash
- Sauerkraut
- White mushrooms
- Portobello mushrooms
- Beetroot
- Brown onion
- Red onion
- Carrots
- Bean sprouts
- Artichoke
- Ginger
- Garlic
- Olives
- Basil
- Sage
- Parsley
- Chives
- Dill

FRUITS AND BERRIES

- Raspberries
- Blackberries
- Strawberries
- Coconut
- Lemon
- Lime
- Starfruit

FATS AND OILS

- Coconut oil
- Olive oil
- Avocado oil
- MCT oil
- Grass fed butter

DAIRY

- Greek yogurt
- Kefir
- Heavy cream
- Half n' Half
- Feta
- Mozzarella
- Cheddar
- Blue cheese
- Parmesan
- Cottage cheese
- Swiss cheese
- Gouda
- Cream cheese
- Colby
- Ricotta
- Brie
- Goat cheese
- Sour cream

DRINKS

- Spring water
- Sparkling water
- Tea
- Coffee
- Bone broth
- Keto greens
- MCT powder mix
- Coconut milk
- Almond milk

CONDIMENTS AND SAUCES

- Apple cider vinegar
- Balsamic vinegar
- Mustard
- Ketchup (sugar free)
- Avocado Mayonnaise
- Salsa
- Lemon juice
- Horseradish
- Lime juice
- Hot sauces
- Soy sauce
- Tabasco

HERBS AND SPICES

- Apple cider vinegar
- Himalayan pink salt
- Sea salt
- Black pepper
- Cilantro
- Cinnamon
- Turmeric
- Cayenne
- Cumin
- Basil
- Thyme
- Sage
- Oregano
- Dill
- Rosemary
- Chili powder
- Paprika

SWEETNERS

- Monk Fruit
- Xylitol
- Lakanto
- Swerve
- Erythritol
- Stevia
- Pyure
- Truvia

CHOCOLATE

- Cocoa Powder
- Cacoa Powder
- Sugar Free Cooking Chocolate
- Dark Chocolate

FLOURS

- Almond Meal
- Almond Flour
- Coconut flour
- Ground Hazelnut flour
- Ground Macadamia flour
- Ground Peanut flour
- Ground Chai Seeds
- Flaxseed Meal
- Sunflower seed meal

THICKENING AGENTS

- Oat Fiber
- Psyllium Husks
- Gelatin
- Glucomannan
- Collagen Protein Powder
- Inulin
- Xanthan gum

ERYTHRITOL	1 TBSP + 1 TSP	1/3 CUP	2/3 CUP	1 1/3 CUP
LIQUID STEVIA	1/16 TSP 6 DROPS	1/4 TSP 24 DROPS	1/2 TSP 48 DROPS	1 TSP 96 DROPS
STEVIA POWDER	1/16 TSP	1/4 TSP	1/2 TSP	1 TSP
TRUVIA ERYTHRITOL + STEVIA	1.5 TSP	1 TBSP + 2 TSP	3.5 TBSP	1/3 CUP + 1.5 TBSP
LIQUID MONK FRUIT	10 DROPS	40 DROPS	80 DROPS	160 DROPS
SWERVE ERYTHRITOL + OLIGOSACHARIDES	1 TBSP	1/4 CUP	1/2 CUP	1 CUP
ALLULOSE	1 TBSP + 1 TSP	5 TBSP + 1 TSP	1/2 CUP + 3 TBSP	1 1/3 CUP
XYLITOL	1 TBSP	1/4 CUP	1/2 CUP	1 CUP

DRY/WEIGHT MEASURE

		OUNCES	POUNDS	METRIC
1/16 TEASPOON	A DASH			
1/8 TEASPOON OR LESS	A PINCH OR 6 DROPS			.5 ML
1/4 TEASPOON	15 DROPS			1 ML
1/2 TEASPOON	30 DROPS			2 ML
1 TEASPOON	1/3 TABLESPOON	1/6 OUNCE		5 ML
3 TEASPOONS	1 TABLESPOON	1/2 OUNCE		14 GR
1 TABLESPOON	3 TEASPOONS	1/2 OUNCE		14 GR
2 TABLESPOONS	1/8 CUP	1 OUNCE		28 GR
4 TABLESPOONS	1/4 CUP	2 OUNCES		56.7 GR
5 TABLESPOONS + 1 TEASPOON	1/3 CUP	2.6 OUNCES		75.6 GR
8 TABLESPOONS	1/2 CUP	4 OUNCES	1/4 POUND	113 GR
10 TABLESPOONS + 2 TEASPOONS	2/3 CUP	5.2 OUNCES		151 GR
12 TABLESPOONS	3/4 CUP	6 OUNCES	.375 POUND	170 GR
16 TABLESPOONS	1 CUP	8 OUNCES	.500 OR 1/2 POUND	225 GR
32 TABLESPOONS	2 CUPS	16 OUNCES	1 POUND	454 GR
64 TABLESPOONS	4 CUPS OR 1 QUART	32 OUNCES	2 POUNDS	907 GR

LIQUID OR VOLUME MEASUREMENTS

JIGGER OR MEASURE	1 1/2 OR 1.5 FLUID OUNCES		3 TABLESPOONS	45 ML
1 CUP	8 FLUID OUNCES	1/2 PINT	16 TABLESPOONS	237 ML
2 CUPS	16 FLUID OUNCES	1 PINT	32 TABLESPOONS	474 ML
4 CUPS	32 FLUID OUNCES	1 QUART	64 TABLESPOONS	946 .4 ML
2 PINTS	32 FLUID OUNCES	1 QUART	4 CUPS	946 ML
4 QUARTS	128 FLUID OUNCES	1 GALLON	16 CUPS	3.785 L
8 QUARTS	256 FLUID OUNCES OR ONE PECK	2 GALLONS	32 CUPS	7.57 L
4 PECKS	ONE BUSHEL			
DASH	LESS THAN 1/4 TEASPOON			

CONVERSIONS FOR INGREDIENTS COMMONLY USED IN BAKING

INGREDIENTS	OUNCES	GRAMS
1 CUP ALL PURPOSE FLOUR	5	142
1 CUP GRANULATED SWEETENER	7	198
1 CUP FIRMLY PACKED SWEETENER	7	198
1 CUP POWDERED (CONFECTIONERS') SWEETENER	4	113
1 CUP COCOA POWDER	3	85
BUTTER (SALTED OR UNSALTED)		
4 TABLESPOONS = 1/2 STICK = 1/4 CUP	2	57
8 TABLESPOONS = 1 STICK = 1/2 CUP	4	113
16 TABLESPOONS = 2 STICKS = 1 CUP	8	227

OVEN TEMPERATURES

FAHRENHEIT (DEGREES)	CELSIUS	GAS MARK (IMPERIAL)	DESCRIPTION
225	105	1/3	VERY COOL
250	120	1/2	
275	130	1	COOL
300	150	2	
325	165	3	VERY MODERATE
350	180	4	MODERATE
375	190	5	
400	200	6	MODERATELY HOT
425	220	7	HOT
450	230	8	
475	245	9	VERY HOT

28 Day
Meal Plan

Welcome to the Ketoveo tribe for your meal planning over the next 28 days. Here you can follow our step-by-step ready-made recipes over the next four weeks. You can also follow your very own creative meal planning ideas with the use of the Ketoveo shopping list and friendly food list to see what meal plans you want to create over the next 28 days.

Let's get you started on your journey into ketosis!

Here are our suggested meal plans, including all recipes, for your next 28 days. Feel free to mix them up however you wish and simply have fun with it!

WEEK ONE

Day 1	Day 2	Day 3	Day 4
BREAKFAST	**BREAKFAST**	**BREAKFAST**	**BREAKFAST**
Spinach, Feta Scrambled Eggs	Almond Cocoa Protein Smoothie	Spinach, Feta Scrambled Eggs	Coconut/Almond Pancakes
LUNCH	**LUNCH**	**LUNCH**	**LUNCH**
Bacon, Avocado & Egg Salad	Sliced Steak with Brussels Sprouts	Lettuce Beef Hamburger	Zesty Prawns & Avocado Salad
DINNER	**DINNER**	**DINNER**	**DINNER**
Garlic Chicken with Broccoli & Spinach	Grilled Salmon with Avocado Salsa	Chicken Taco Lettuce Wraps	Garlic Chicken with Broccoli & Spinach

Day 5	Day 6	Day 7	
BREAKFAST	**BREAKFAST**	**BREAKFAST**	
Omelet with Onions, Peppers & Cheese	Almond Cocoa Protein Smoothie	Omelet with Onions, Peppers & Cheese	
LUNCH	**LUNCH**	**LUNCH**	
Bacon, Avocado & Egg Salad	Lettuce Beef Hamburger	Zesty Prawns & Avocado Salad	
DINNER	**DINNER**	**DINNER**	
Grilled Salmon with Avocado Salsa	Garlic Prawn Courgette Pasta	Chicken Taco Lettuce Wraps	

WEEK TWO

Day 8	Day 9	Day 10	Day 11
BREAKFAST	BREAKFAST	BREAKFAST	BREAKFAST
Coconut/Almond Pancakes	Omelet with Onions, Peppers & Cheese	Avocado Mint Green Smoothie	Yogurt, Almond Butter, Raspberries & Coconut
LUNCH	LUNCH	LUNCH	LUNCH
Lettuce Beef Hamburger	Zesty Prawns & Avocado Salad	Chicken Wings, Celery Sticks & Nut Dip	Cutlets Marinated in Red Pesto
DINNER	DINNER	DINNER	DINNER
Garlic Prawn Courgette Pasta	Chicken Taco Lettuce Wraps	Garlic Steak Bites	Sesame Salmon with Baby Pak Choi & Mushrooms

Day 12	Day 13	Day 14	
BREAKFAST	BREAKFAST	BREAKFAST	
Avocado Mint Green Smoothie	Yogurt, Almond Butter, Raspberries & Coconut	Avocado Mint Green Smoothie	
LUNCH	LUNCH	LUNCH	
Lettuce Beef Hamburger	Chicken Wings, Celery Sticks & Nut Dip	Cutlet Marinated in Red Pesto	
DINNER	DINNER	DINNER	
Pesto Chicken & Veggies	Sesame Salmon with Baby Pak Choi & Mushrooms	Garlic Steak Bites	

WEEK THREE

Day 15	Day 16	Day 17	Day 18
BREAKFAST	BREAKFAST	BREAKFAST	BREAKFAST
Almond Cocoa Protein Smoothie	Boiled Eggs & Avocado	Yogurt, Almond Butter, Raspberries & Coconut	Coconut Almond Hot Cereal
LUNCH	LUNCH	LUNCH	LUNCH
Avocado Tuna Salad	Cutlets Marinated in Red Pesto	Zesty Prawns & Avocado Salad	Avocado Tuna Salad
DINNER	DINNER	DINNER	DINNER
Sesame Salmon with Baby Pak Choi & Mushrooms	Pesto Chicken & Veggies	Stir-Fry Chicken & Veggies	Thai Coconut Soup

Day 19	Day 20	Day 21	
BREAKFAST	BREAKFAST	BREAKFAST	
Almond Cocoa Protein Smoothie	Boiled Eggs & Avocado	Coconut Almond Hot Cereal	
LUNCH	LUNCH	LUNCH	
Cutlets Marinated in Red Pesto	Zesty Prawns & Avocado Salad	Caesar Salad	
DINNER	DINNER	DINNER	
Lemon Garlic Steak	Stir-Fry Chicken & Veggies	Garlic Prawn Courgette Pasta	

WEEK FOUR

Day 22	Day 23	Day 24	Day 25
BREAKFAST	BREAKFAST	BREAKFAST	BREAKFAST
Fried Eggs & Crispy Bacon	Almond Cocoa Protein Smoothie	Fried Eggs with Avocado	Avocado Mint Green Smoothie
LUNCH	LUNCH	LUNCH	LUNCH
Garlic Chicken Courgetti	Cutlets Marinated in Red Pesto	Garlic Chicken Courgetti	Salmon & Broccoli Saute
DINNER	DINNER	DINNER	DINNER
Garlic Steak Bites	Stir-Fry Chicken & Veggies	Garlic Prawn Courgette Pasta	Pesto Chicken & Veggies

Day 26	Day 27	Day 28	
BREAKFAST	BREAKFAST	BREAKFAST	
Fried Eggs & Crispy Bacon	Yogurt, Almond Butter, Raspberries & Coconut	Fried Eggs with Avocado	
LUNCH	LUNCH	LUNCH	
Caesar Salad	Cutlets Marinated in Red Pesto	Salmon & Broccoli Saute	
DINNER	DINNER	DINNER	
Thai Coconut Soup	Lemon Garlic Steak	Thai Coconut Soup	

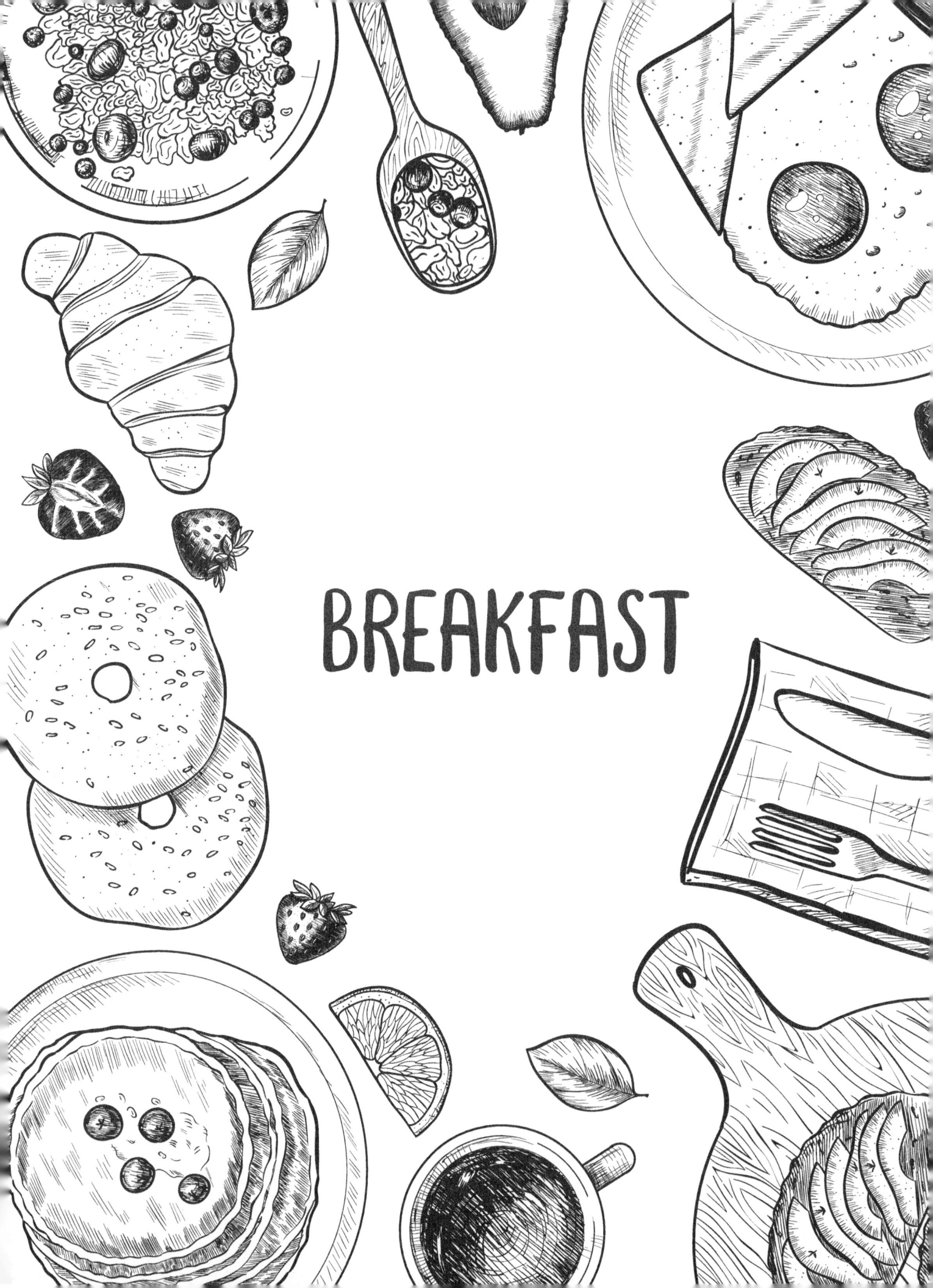

BREAKFAST

BREAKFAST MENU

Spinach Feta Scrambled Eggs - 60

Almond Cocoa Protein Smoothie - 61

Coconut / Almond Pancakes - 62

Omelet with Onions, Peppers & Cheese - 63

Avocado Mint Green Smoothie - 64

Yogurt, Almond Butter, Raspberries & Coconut - 65

Boiled Eggs & Avocado - 66

Coconut Almond Hot Cereal - 67

Fried Eggs & Crispy Bacon - 68

Fried Eggs With Avocado - 69

SPINACH FETA SCRAMBLED EGGS

Servings: 1		Time: 7 min
Nutritional Facts Per Serving:		
Net Carbs:	4.6 g	Protein:	30.4 g
Fat:	35.5 g	Calories:	458 kcal

Ingredients:

3 large eggs
1 cup spinach leaves, washed
½ cup feta cheese
Salt & black pepper
Drizzle of coconut oil

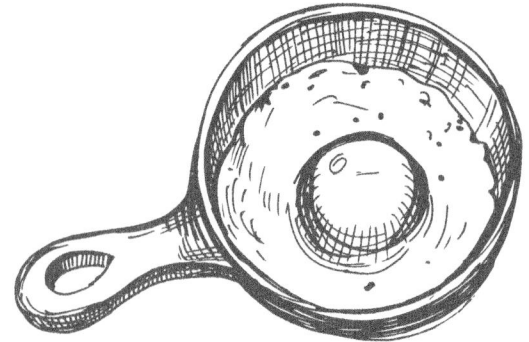

THIS IS HOW YOU MAKE THE RECIPE

1. Heat up a frying pan with a drizzle coconut oil on low-medium heat.
2. Whilst your pan is heating up. Grab a bowl and crack 3 eggs into it, add your spinach, feta, salt and pepper.
3. Whisk all together and pour into the pan.
4. Scramble them up, serve when ready.

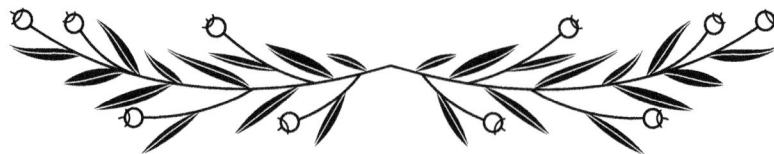

ALMOND COCOA PROTEIN SMOOTHIE

Servings: 1		Time: 5 min	
Nutritional Facts Per Serving:			
Net Carbs:	6.8 g	Protein:	35 g
Fat:	44 g	Calories:	575 kcal

Ingredients:

2 tbsp natural almond butter
1 tbsp unsweetened cocoa powder
2 cups unsweetened almond milk
2 tbsp full-fat yogurt
1 large egg
Optional: sweetener to taste

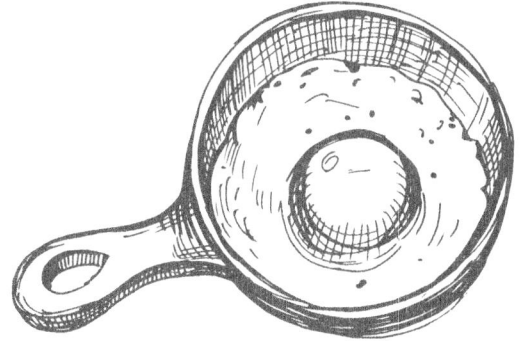

THIS IS HOW YOU MAKE THE RECIPE

1. Pour the almond milk, yogurt, egg, almond butter, cocoa and optional sweetener into the blender and blend until well mixed.
2. Serve and enjoy!

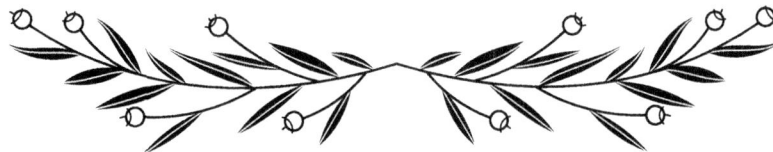

COCONUT / ALMOND PANCAKES

COCONUT PANCAKES

Servings: 5		Time: 30 min	
Nutritional Facts Per Serving:			
Net Carbs:	2.6 g	Protein:	6.8 g
Fat:	17.6 g	Calories:	198 kcal

ALMOND PANCAKES

Servings: 9		Time: 30 min	
Nutritional Facts Per Serving:			
Carbs:	2.2 g	Protein:	5.9 g
Fat:	11.6 g	Calories:	142.4 kcal

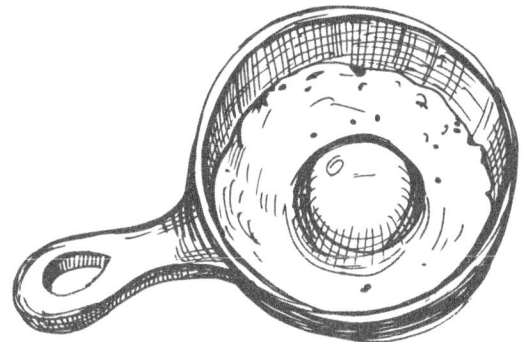

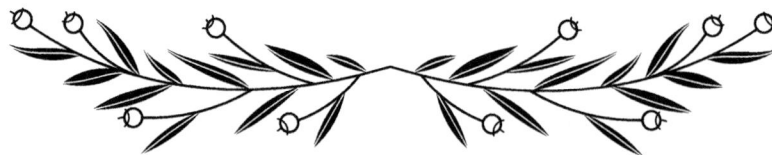

Ingredients:

Coconut oil
¾ cup almond flour or ¼ cup coconut flour
4 large eggs
½ cup soft white cheese (cream cheese)
Vanilla extract, to taste
Pinch of cinnamon
1 tbsp sweetener
1 tsp baking powder

THIS IS HOW YOU MAKE THE RECIPE

1. Put the cream cheese into a bowl that is safe to microwave for about 10 seconds to make it soft.
2. Add in the rest of the ingredients and whisk until smooth. Let it settle for 10 minutes.
3. Use ¼ cup to make sure they are all the same in size, cook them in some coconut oil on low heat as these brown quickly.
4. You can add cocoa, raspberries, strawberries or pumpkin spices etc. into the mix for more variety.

OMELET WITH ONIONS, PEPPERS & CHEESE

Servings: 1		Time: 10 min	
Nutritional Facts Per Serving:			
Net Carbs:	7.4 g	Protein:	48 g
Fat:	76.2 g	Calories:	904 kcal

Ingredients:

3 large eggs
1 tbsp whipping cream
1 slice onion, chopped
½ slice sweet pepper: red, yellow, green or orange
1 cup cheddar cheese, grated
Salt & black pepper
Drizzle of coconut oil

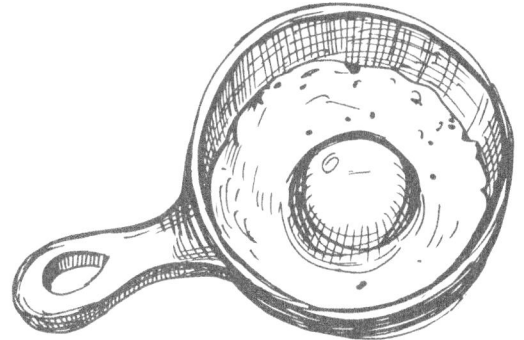

THIS IS HOW YOU MAKE THE RECIPE

1. Heat up your pan with a drizzle of coconut oil on low-medium heat.
2. Get a mixing bowl and crack the eggs, cream, onion, pepper, salt and black pepper all in.
3. Whisk it all together until it's fluffy. Pour mixture into the pan, after 2 minutes sprinkle your cheese on top.
4. When ready, fold half of the omelet over and serve.

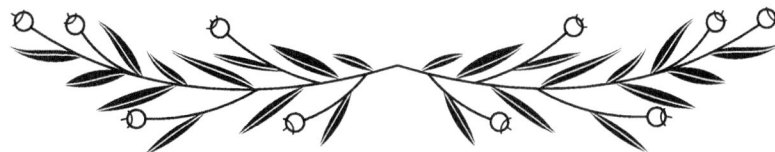

AVOCADO MINT GREEN SMOOTHIE

Servings: 1   Time: 5 min

Nutritional Facts Per Serving:

Net Carbs:	3.4 g	Protein:	2.6 g
Fat:	24.4 g	Calories:	264 kcal

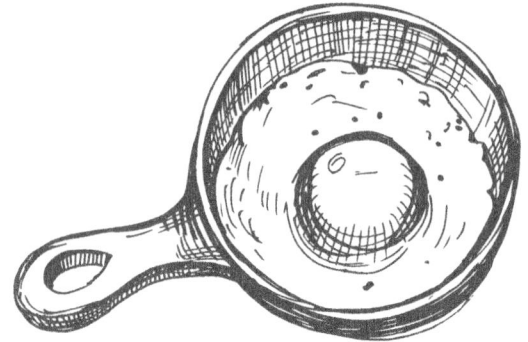

Ingredients:

½ avocado

¾ cup unsweetened coconut milk

½ cup almond milk

Sweetener to taste

5-6 large mint leaves

3 sprigs of coriander

1 squeeze of lime juice

¼ tsp vanilla extract

THIS IS HOW YOU MAKE THE RECIPE

1. Place all of the ingredients into the blender. Blend on low speed until completely pureed.

2. Taste to adjust sweetness and tartness.

3. Serve and enjoy.

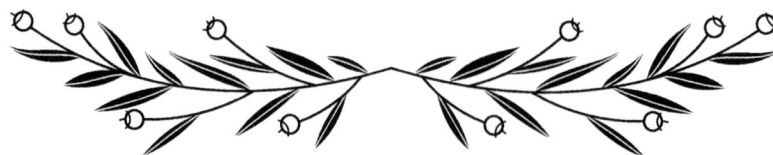

YOGURT, ALMOND BUTTER, RASPBERRY & COCONUT

Servings: 1		Time: 2 min
Nutritional Facts Per Serving:		
Net Carbs:	14.7 g	Protein:	25.7 g
Fat.	31.4 g	Calories:	442 kcal

Ingredients:

1 cup of full fat yogurt
1 tbsp natural almond butter
¼ cup raspberries
1 tbsp unsweetened coconut flakes

THIS IS HOW YOU MAKE THE RECIPE

1. Pour yogurt into a bowl, add almond butter and mix together.
2. Then add your raspberries and coconut flakes.
3. Eat and enjoy!

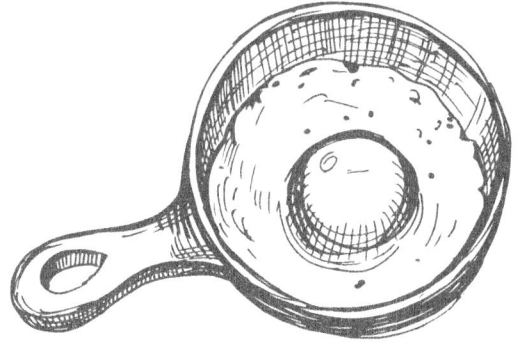

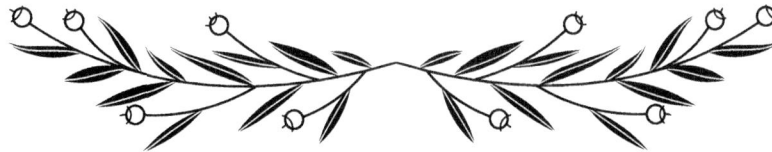

BOILED EGGS & AVOCADO

Servings: 1	Time: 8 min
Nutritional Facts Per Serving:	
Net Carbs: 3.2 g	Protein: 15 g
Fat: 44 g	Calories: 489 kcal

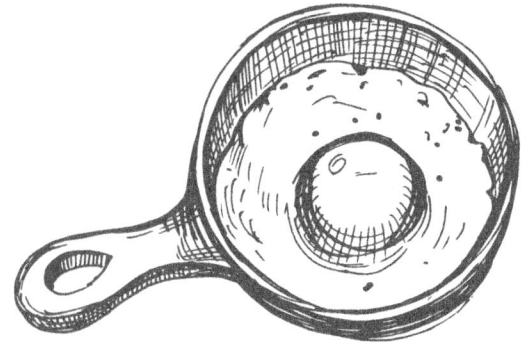

Ingredients:

2 large eggs

1 avocado

Salt & black pepper

Drizzle of olive oil

THIS IS HOW YOU MAKE THE RECIPE

1. Boil two eggs, 5 minutes for a more runny egg or 7 minutes for a harder egg.
2. Cut an avocado in half, remove pip and scoop out each half with a spoon.
3. Peel eggs once cooled, add each egg into the hole of each avocado.

4. Add salt and pepper and enjoy!

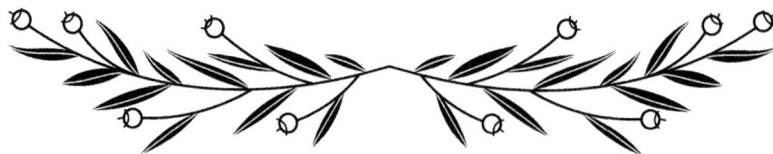

COCONUT ALMOND HOT CEREAL

Servings: 1		Time: 7 min	
Nutritional Facts Per Serving:			
Net Carbs:	5.2 g	Protein:	11 g
Fat:	50 g	Calories:	521 kcal

Ingredients:

2 tbsp ground almond/almond meal

2 tbsp ground flaxseed /linseed meal

2 tbsp unsweetened coconut flakes

1 pinch of salt

1 tbsp natural almond butter

⅓ cup boiling water

¼ cup double cream or coconut milk

Optional: sweetener to taste

THIS IS HOW YOU MAKE THE RECIPE

1. In a bowl mix all the dry ingredients together, add 1 tablespoon of almond butter and boiling water.

2. Mix all together. Cover the bowl to sit for 2-3 minutes.

3. Add ¼ cup of double cream or coconut milk. Add optional sweetener to taste.

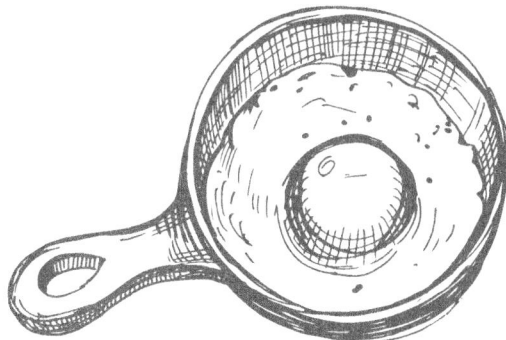

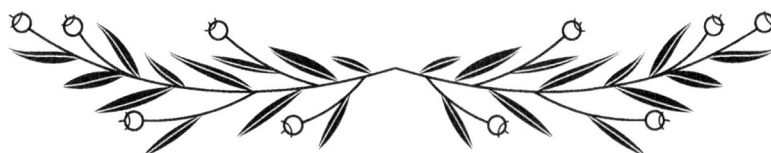

4. Stir and enjoy!

FRIED EGGS & CRISPY BACON

Servings: 1		Time: 10 min	
Nutritional Facts Per Serving:			
Net Carbs:	3.22 g	Protein:	15 g
Fat:	44 g	Calories:	396 kcal

Ingredients:

3 large eggs
3 bacon strips
Salt & black pepper

THIS IS HOW YOU MAKE THE RECIPE

1. Heat a pan on low-medium heat, when heated cook the bacon on both sides until it's done according to how you like it.

2. Once the bacon is done, crack your 3 eggs into the pan and cook until ready to serve.

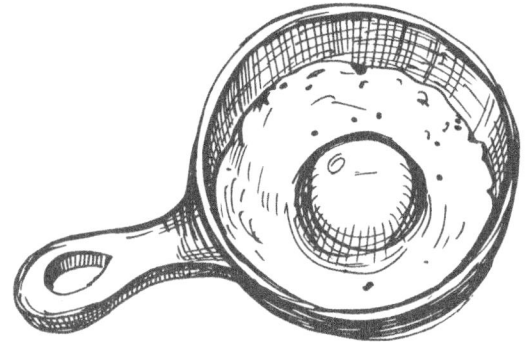

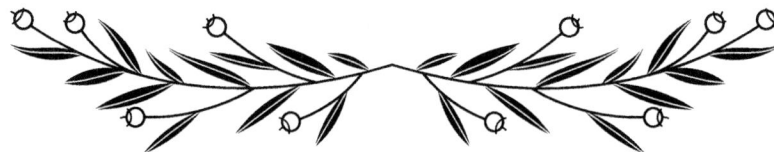

3. Enjoy!

FRIED EGGS WITH AVOCADO

Servings: 1		Time: 8 min	
Nutritional Facts Per Serving:			
Net Carbs:	4.4 g	Protein:	16.5 g
Fat:	57.6 g	Calories:	627 kcal

Ingredients:

1 avocado
2 large eggs
Drizzle of olive oil

THIS IS HOW YOU MAKE THE RECIPE

1. Heat a pan on low to medium heat with some olive oil.
2. Slice your avocado in half, remove seed and carefully scoop out the avocado halves. Now slice each half of your avocado so it has a hole in the center of each slice.
3. Use these two slices to put into the pan and crack open each egg to place in the middle of the avocado holes to fry until ready to serve.
4. Use the leftover avocado to add to your meal and enjoy!

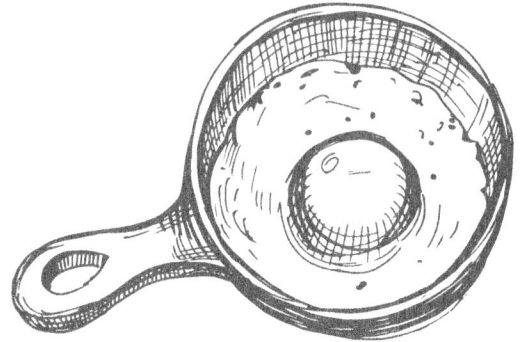

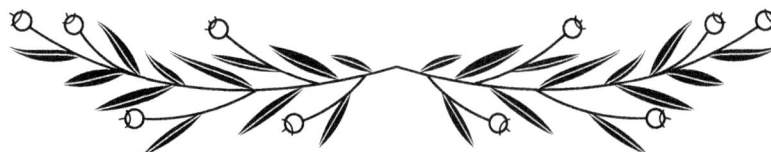

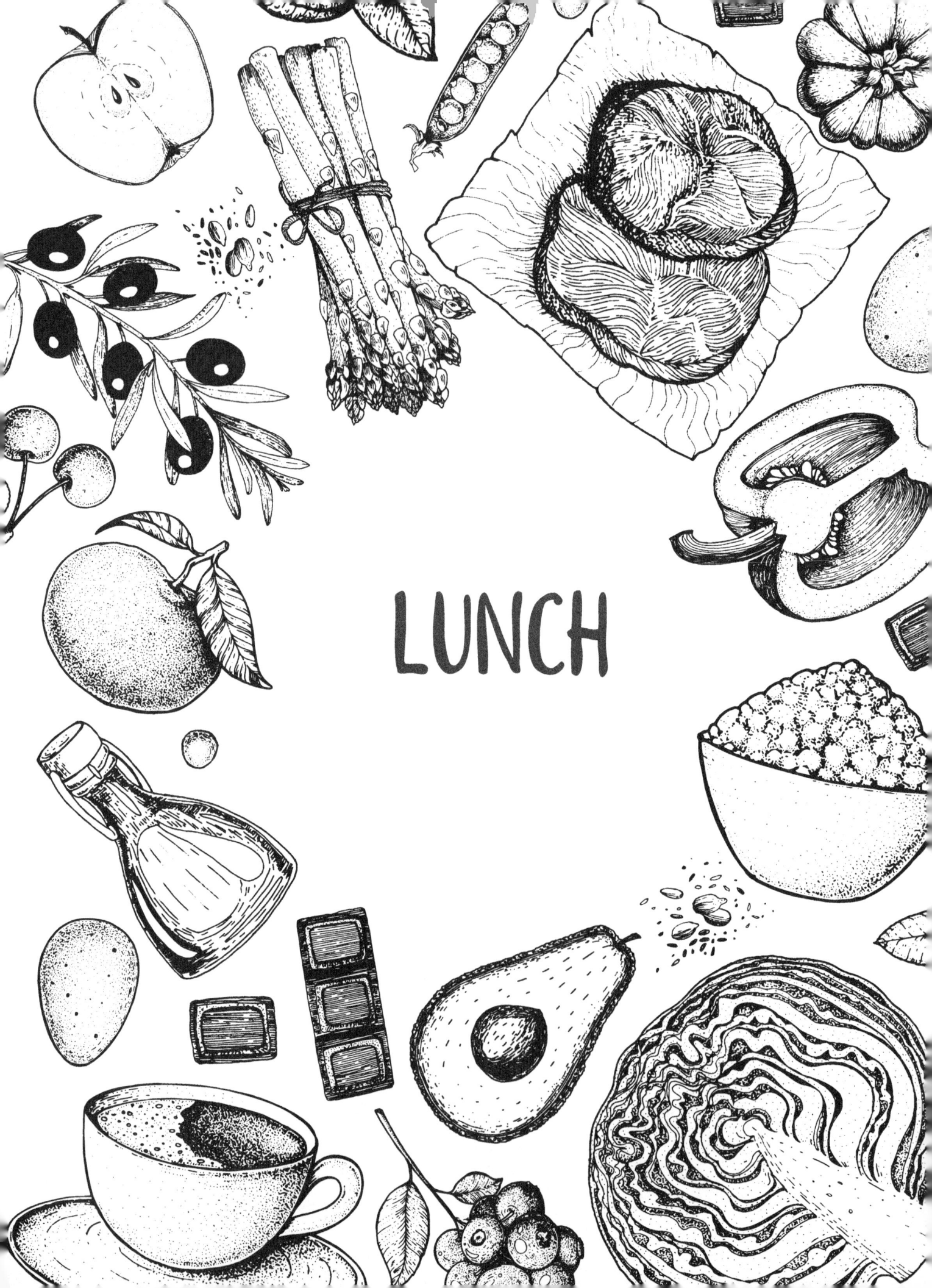

LUNCH

LUNCH MENU

Bacon, Avocado & Egg Salad - 72

Sliced Steak with Brussels Sprouts - 73

Lettuce Beef Hamburger - 74

Zesty Lime Prawns & Avocado Salad - 75

Chicken Wings, Celery Sticks & Nut Dip - 76

Cutlets Marinated in Red Pesto - 77

Avocado Tuna Salad - 78

Caesar Salad - 79

Garlic Chicken Courgetti - 80

Salmon & Broccoli Saute - 81

BACON, AVOCADO & EGG SALAD

Servings: 1		Time: 10 min	
Nutritional Facts Per Serving:			
Net Carbs:	6.5 g	Protein:	33 g
Fat:	64 g	Calories:	766 kcal

Ingredients:

3 bacon strips
1 avocado
2 large eggs
Bowl of lettuce
½ cucumber
¼ cup feta cheese
Drizzle of olive oil
Squeeze of lemon

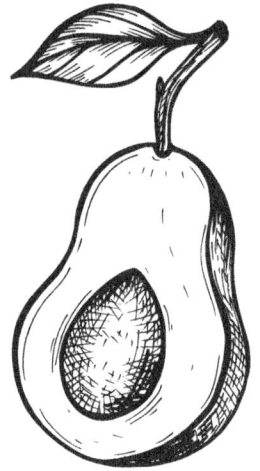

THIS IS HOW YOU MAKE THE RECIPE

1. Heat a pan on low-medium heat and cook your bacon until crispy.
2. Heat up a small pot of water and add your eggs to boil for 5-7 minutes.
3. Wash and chop up the lettuce and cucumber into a bowl.
4. Sprinkle some feta on top.
5. After your eggs are boiled let them cool down. Peel and cut them up into quarters to put into your salad.
6. Take your bacon when cooled after cooking and place them into your salad.
7. Add a drizzle of olive oil and squeeze some lemon for some flavour.

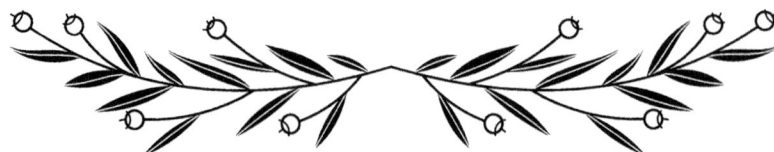

SLICED STEAK WITH BRUSSELS SPROUTS

Servings: 1   Time: 35 min

Nutritional Facts Per Serving:
Net Carbs: 8.47 g   Protein: 230 g
Fat: 188 g   Calories: 2705 kcal

Ingredients:

3 tbsp butter
2 spring onions, chopped
1 medium skirt steak, cut into 4 slices
½ tsp salt
¼ tsp black pepper
1 cup Brussels sprouts, cut in half
1½ tsp olive oil

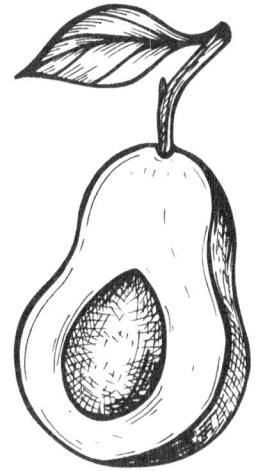

THIS IS HOW YOU MAKE THE RECIPE

1. Preheat a large cast-iron pan on high heat.
2. Meanwhile, in a small bowl, whip butter and chopped up spring onions. Set aside.
3. Rinse and pat dry the steak with a paper towel. Season generously with salt and pepper.
4. When the cast-iron pan is hot, add ½ teaspoon olive oil to the pan and the sliced steak. Sear on high for 3 minutes each side.
5. Add ½ tablespoon of spring onion butter over each steak. Cover loosely with foil and let rest.
6. In a mixing bowl, combine Brussels sprouts and 1 tablespoon olive oil. Season with ½ teaspoon salt and ¼ teaspoon pepper.
7. In the same pan, sear Brussels sprouts on the cut side down until golden brown, about 5 minutes.
8. If you want a crispier texture, add more olive oil and cook for a few more minutes.
9. Serve with remaining butter and enjoy!

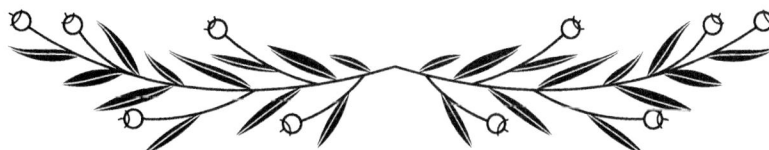

LETTUCE BEEF HAMBURGER

Servings: 1		Time: 20 min
Nutritional Facts Per Serving:		
Net Carbs:	3 g	Protein: 29 g
Fat:	45 g	Calories: 551 kcal

Ingredients:

1 beef burger
1 large iceberg lettuce leaf
1 slice tomato
1-2 slices cheddar cheese
½ avocado, sliced
Salt & black pepper
2 sprigs of coriander
Drizzle of olive oil

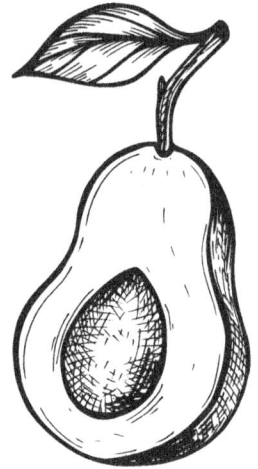

THIS IS HOW YOU MAKE THE RECIPE

1. Heat up a pan at medium heat with some olive oil and place your beef burger in. Flip over once it is crispy brown.
2. Wash the lettuce leaf and place it on your plate, when both sides of your beef burger are cooked place it in the lettuce leaf bowl.
3. Place your sliced tomato, sliced cheese, avocado and coriander on top. Add salt and pepper to your liking and enjoy!

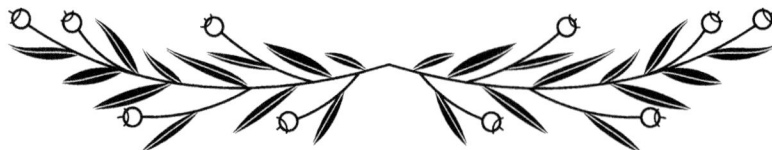

ZESTY LIME PRAWNS & AVOCADO SALAD

Servings: 4		Time: 10 min	
Nutritional Facts Per Serving:			
Net Carbs:	3 g	Protein:	2.75 g
Fat:	8.5 g	Calories:	224 kcal

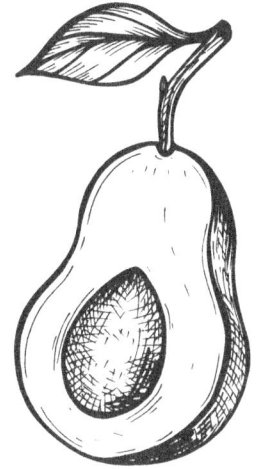

Ingredients:

¼ cup red onion, chopped

2 small limes, juiced

1 tsp olive oil

¼ tsp salt

Black pepper

500g peeled prawns, cooked & cut into bite-size pieces

1 medium avocado, chopped

1 medium tomato, chopped

1 fresh jalapeno pepper, seeded & finely chopped

1 tbsp fresh coriander, chopped

THIS IS HOW YOU MAKE THE RECIPE

1. In a small bowl, combine the onion, lime juice, olive oil, salt, and pepper to taste. Let it sit for at least 5 minutes.
2. In a large bowl, combine the prawns, avocado, tomato, and jalapeno.
3. Add the onion mixture and the coriander, and toss gently.
4. Season with pepper, if desired and enjoy!

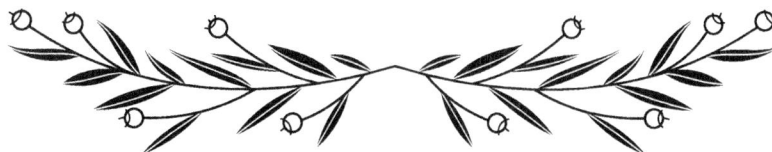

CHICKEN WINGS, CELERY STICKS & NUT DIP

Servings: 2		Time: 45 min
Nutritional Facts Per Serving:		
Net Carbs:	3 g	Protein:	85 g
Fat:	80 g	Calories:	1095 kcal

Ingredients:

6 chicken wing segments, flats & drums
2 tbsp olive oil
3 tsp all purpose seasoning of your choice
2 celery sticks, washed
2 tbsp natural almond butter

THIS IS HOW YOU MAKE THE RECIPE

1. Preheat the oven to 390°F.
2. Line a baking tray with foil and then place a cooling rack inside the baking tray.
3. In a small bowl combine the olive oil and seasoning, stir till combined.
4. Pat the chicken wing segments dry with some paper towel and place them in a large bowl.
5. Pour the seasoned olive oil over the chicken segments and toss until they are all completely coated. Use your hands if needed.
6. Place the wings on the rack over the tray, space them evenly so the air can circulate around them.
7. Place in the oven for 40-45 minutes until they are golden brown and the skin is crispy.
8. Serve with your sliced celery sticks and almond butter as a dip.

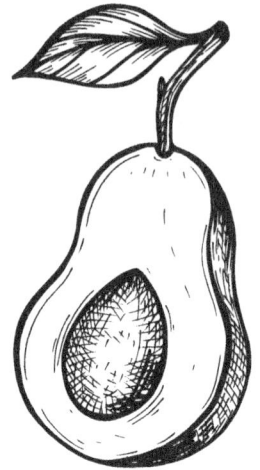

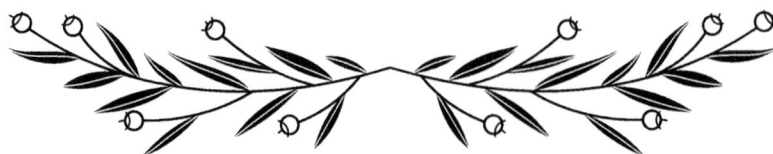

CUTLETS MARINATED IN RED PESTO

Servings: 1	Time: 15 min

Nutritional Facts Per Serving:
Net Carbs: 3.7 g Protein: 42 g
Fat: 50 g Calories: 634 kcal

Ingredients:

1 pork cutlet
½ tbsp butter or olive oil
1 tbsp red pesto

Pesto mayonnaise:
2 tbsp keto friendly mayonnaise
½ tbsp red pesto

Salad:
½ cup broccoli florets, washed
½ cup cauliflower florets, washed
¼ cup cheese, grated
¼ cup rocket, washed

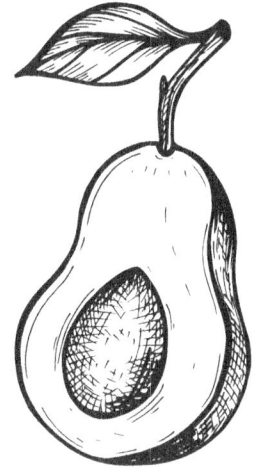

THIS IS HOW YOU MAKE THE RECIPE

1. Rub the pork cutlet with pesto and fry on medium heat in butter or oil for 8 minutes. Let simmer for 4 more minutes on low heat.
2. Mix mayonnaise with red pesto. Serve on the side.
3. Mix your broccoli, cauliflower and rocket with grated cheese for the salad.
4. Serve and enjoy!

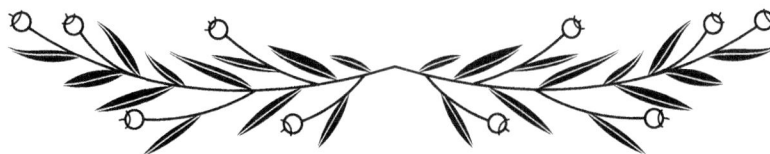

AVOCADO TUNA SALAD

Servings: 4	Time: 10 min
Nutritional Facts Per Serving:	
Net Carbs: 2.6 g	Protein: 10.5 g
Fat: 10 g	Calories: 152 kcal

Ingredients:

1 tin tuna, drain water or oil
1 avocado, chopped
½ cup cucumber, chopped
¼ cup celery, finely chopped
¼ cup onion, finely chopped
2 tbsp fresh coriander or parsley, chopped
1 tbsp olive oil
1 tbsp lemon juice
½ tsp salt
Black pepper

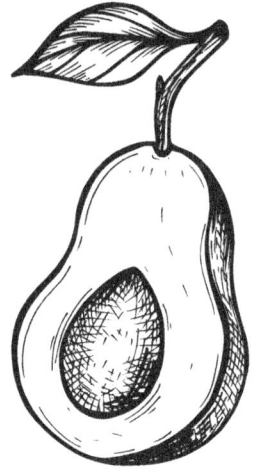

THIS IS HOW YOU MAKE THE RECIPE

1. Place all of the ingredients in a medium bowl.
2. Mix with a fork or spoon until the avocado is roughly mashed and mixed through.
3. Serve on lettuce wraps and enjoy!

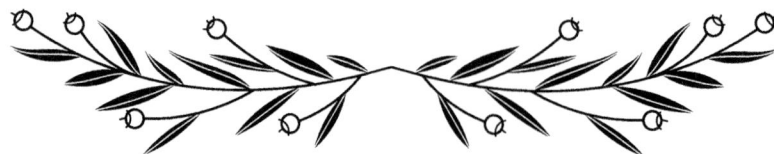

CAESAR SALAD

Servings: 2   Time: 30 min

Nutritional Facts Per Serving:
Net Carbs: 6.3 g   Protein: 66 g
Fat: 28 g   Calories: 558 kcal

Ingredients:

2 medium chicken breasts, boneless & skinless
1 tbsp olive oil
Salt & black pepper
4 bacon strips
4 cups Cos lettuce, washed & shredded
2 tbsp Parmesan cheese, grated

Dressing:
1 tbsp Dijon mustard
½ lemon, zest & juice
2 tbsp Parmesan cheese, grated
2 tbsp fillets of anchovies, finely chopped
Salt & black pepper
Optional: 1 garlic clove, pressed or finely chopped

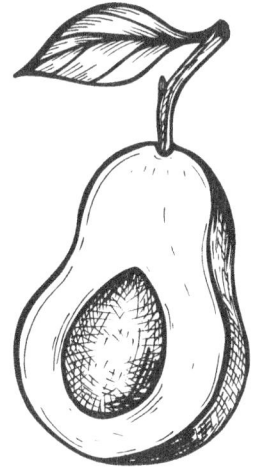

THIS IS HOW YOU MAKE THE RECIPE

1. Preheat the oven to 400°F.
2. Mix the ingredients for the dressing with a whisk or an immersion blender. Set aside in the refrigerator.
3. Place the chicken breasts in a greased baking dish. Season the chicken with salt, pepper and drizzle with olive oil or melted butter on top.
4. Bake the chicken in the oven for about 20 minutes or until fully cooked through. You can also cook the chicken on the stove top if you prefer.
5. In a pan, fry the bacon until crisp.
6. Once the chicken is cooked, slice each breast up.
7. Place the washed and shredded lettuce between two plates. Then place the sliced chicken with the crispy, crumbled bacon on top of each plate of lettuce.
8. Finish with a generous dollop of dressing and grated Parmesan cheese.

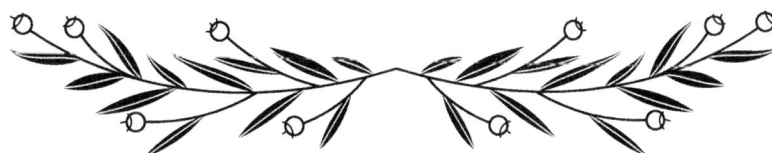

GARLIC CHICKEN COURGETTI

Servings: 2		Time: 15 min	
Nutritional Facts Per Serving:			
Net Carbs:	11 g	Protein:	41 g
Fat:	19 g	Calories:	376 kcal

Ingredients:

2 medium chicken breasts, cut into ½-inch pieces
2 tbsp olive oil
4 garlic cloves, minced or crushed
3 courgettes, spiralized
5 broccoli florets, washed
Salt & black pepper
Optional: ½ tsp red pepper flakes

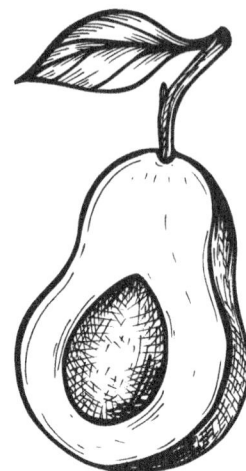

THIS IS HOW YOU MAKE THE RECIPE

1. Heat a large cast-iron pan to medium-high heat. Add olive oil and minced garlic.
2. Cook garlic for 30 seconds to a minute.
3. Add chicken, red pepper flakes (optional), salt and pepper.
4. Cook the chicken for 3 minutes and then add the broccoli to cook with the chicken for another 5 minutes. Turn the chicken over half way through to cook through both sides until golden.
5. Toss in courgetti (courgette spaghetti) and cook for 1 extra minute then turn off heat.
6. Sprinkle with Parmesan cheese if desired, serve and enjoy!

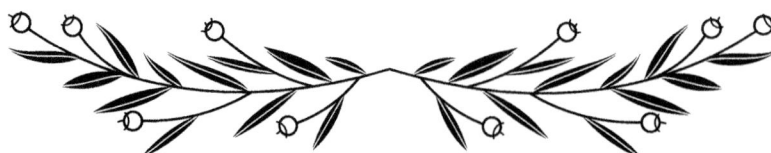

SALMON & BROCCOLI SAUTE

Servings: 4		Time: 10 min	
Nutritional Facts Per Serving:			
Net Carbs:	3.17 g	Protein:	71 g
Fat:	54 g	Calories:	807 kcal

Ingredients:

4 tbsp avocado oil

6 garlic cloves, minced or finely diced

2 tbsp fresh ginger, finely diced

4 eggs, whisked

1 head of broccoli, chopped small

4 salmon fillets, diced

Salt & black pepper

Optional: 2 tbsp tamari sauce/coconut aminos

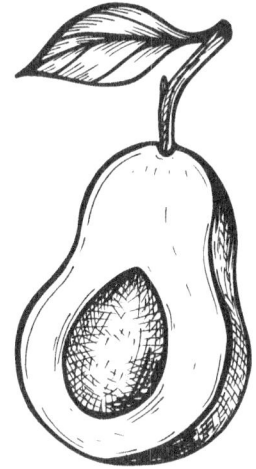

THIS IS HOW YOU MAKE THE RECIPE

1. In a large pan over medium-high heat, add the avocado oil.

2. Add garlic and ginger to the pan. Sauté until fragrant, about 30 seconds.

3. Add the eggs to the pan and cook for about 1-2 minutes.

4. Add the broccoli to the pan and cook until slightly softened, about 5-6 minutes.

5. Add the salmon and optional coconut aminos/tamari sauce to the pan and sauté until the salmon is cooked through, about 2-4 minutes.

6. Season with salt and pepper, to taste and enjoy!

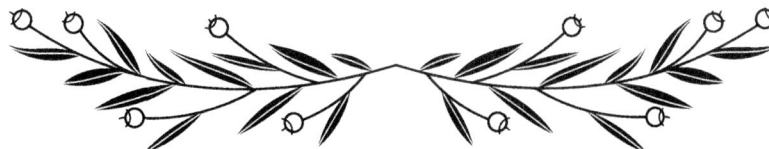

DINNER

DINNER MENU

Garlic Chicken with Broccoli & Spinach - 84

Grilled Salmon with Avocado & Salsa - 85

Chicken Taco Lettuce Wraps - 86

Garlic Prawn Courgette Pasta - 87

Garlic Steak Bites - 88

Sesame Salmon with Baby Pak choi & Mushrooms - 89

Pesto Chicken & Veggies - 90

Stir -Fry Chicken & Veggies - 91

Thai Chicken Soup - 92

Lemon Garlic Steak - 93

GARLIC CHICKEN WITH BROCCOLI & SPINACH

Servings: 4	Time: 15 min
Nutritional Facts Per Serving:	
Net Carbs: 6.7 g	Protein: 42 g
Fat: 24.24 g	Calories: 430 kcal

Ingredients:

454g chicken breasts. cut into 1-inch pieces
2 tbsp olive oil
1 tsp Italian seasoning
Salt & black pepper
3-4 garlic cloves, minced
½ cup red sweet peppers, chopped
2 cups broccoli florets
2 cups baby spinach
½ cup cheddar/mozzarella cheese, grated
½ cup soft white cheese (cream cheese)

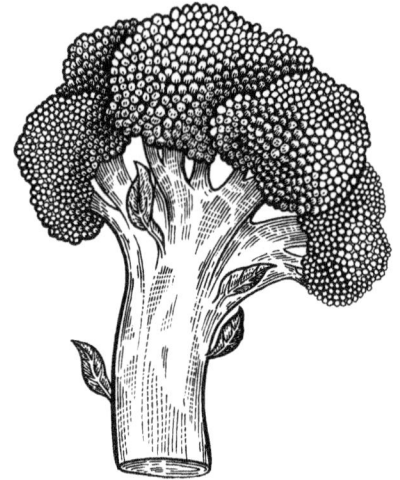

THIS IS HOW YOU MAKE THE RECIPE

1. Heat 2 tablespoons of olive oil in a large saucepan over medium-high heat.
2. Add chopped chicken breasts, season with Italian seasoning, crushed red pepper, salt and pepper. Sauté for 4-5 minutes or until chicken is golden and cooked through.
3. Add the garlic and sauté for another minute.
4. Add the red peppers, broccoli, spinach, shredded cheese, and cream cheese. Cook for another 3-4 minutes or until the broccoli is cooked through.
5. Serve with cooked courgette noodles or cauliflower rice if you wish.

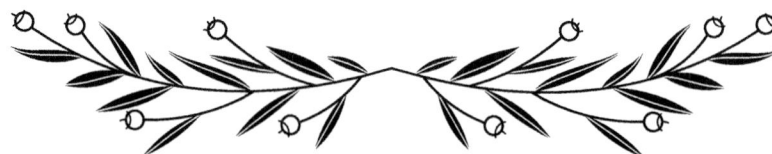

GRILLED SALMON WITH AVOCADO & SALSA

Servings: 2		Time: 10 min	
Nutritional Facts Per Serving:			
Net Carbs:	5.4 g	Protein:	52 g
Fat:	59 g	Calories:	785 kcal

Ingredients:

2 salmon fillets
2 tbsp olive oil
1 garlic clove, minced or crushed
½ tsp chili powder
½ tsp cumin
½ tsp onion powder
¼ tsp black pepper
¼ tsp salt

Avocado salsa:
1 avocado, diced
½ cup tomato, diced
2 tbsp onion, diced
2 tbsp coriander, diced
1 tbsp olive oil
1 tbsp lime juice
Salt & black pepper

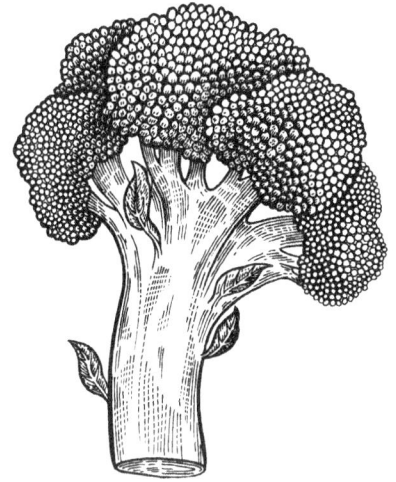

THIS IS HOW YOU MAKE THE RECIPE

1. Heat a large non-stick pan on medium heat.
2. Stir the olive oil, garlic, and spices in a small bowl.
3. Brush or rub salmon with the spice mixture.
4. Add salmon to the pan and cook for 5-6 minutes with the lid on, until the salmon is cooked through.
5. Meanwhile mix all the avocado salsa ingredients together in a small bowl until combined.
6. Remove salmon from pan, top with avocado salsa and serve immediately.

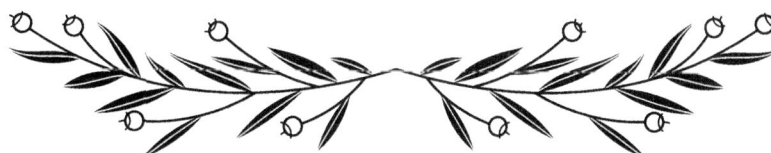

CHICKEN TACO LETTUCE WRAPS

Servings: 4	Time: 30 min
Nutritional Facts Per Serving:	
Net Carbs: 7.5 g	Protein: 40 g
Fat: 19.75 g	Calories: 388 kcal

Ingredients:

Grilled Taco Chicken:
454g chicken breasts or thighs, boneless & skinless
2 tbsp taco seasoning
2 garlic cloves, minced
1 tbsp olive oil

To Assemble:
8 Cos lettuce leaves, rinsed
1 avocado, diced
1 tomato, diced
¼ cup onion, diced

Coriander Sauce:
½ cup coriander, loosely packed
½ cup Greek yogurt /soured cream
2 tbsp olive oil
1 garlic clove, minced
½ lime's juice
Pinch of salt
Optional: 1 jalapeno

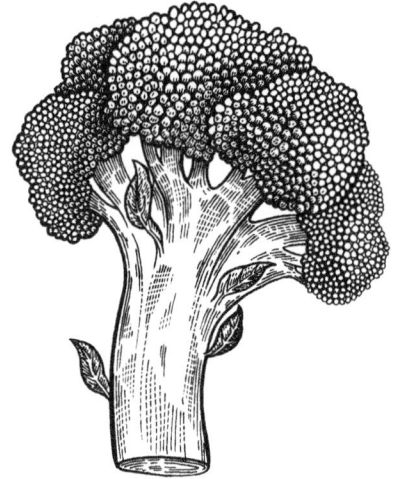

THIS IS HOW YOU MAKE THE RECIPE

1. To cook the chicken add the chicken, garlic, olive oil, and spices in a large bowl or zip-seal bag. Place in the fridge and let marinate for at least 15-30 minutes or up to 24 hours.
2. Remove chicken from marinade and discard the rest.
3. Place chicken on a grill or pan heated to medium-high heat. Let chicken cook until it is no longer pink on the inside, about 7 minutes.
4. To make the coriander sauce, place all the ingredients in the food processor and blend for 1 minute or until creamy.
5. Layer lettuce wraps with chicken, tomatoes, onion, and avocado.
6. Drizzle with coriander sauce or your favorite taco sauce.

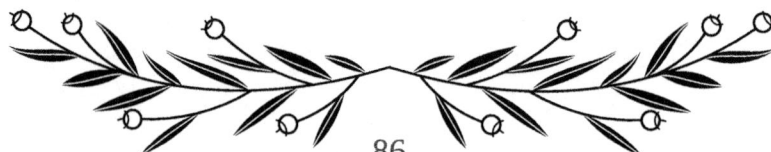

GARLIC PRAWN COURGETTE PASTA

Servings: 4   Time: 15 min

Nutritional Facts Per Serving:
Net Carbs: 5.8 g   Protein: 18.5 g
Fat: 11.5 g   Calories: 204 kcal

Ingredients:

3-4 medium courgette
500g raw prawns, peeled & deveined
1 tbsp olive oil
2 tbsp butter
3-4 garlic cloves, minced or crushed
1 tsp Italian seasoning or oregano
¼ tsp of red pepper flakes, adjust to taste
Salt & black pepper
Optional: Parmesan and parsley, chopped or grated for garnish

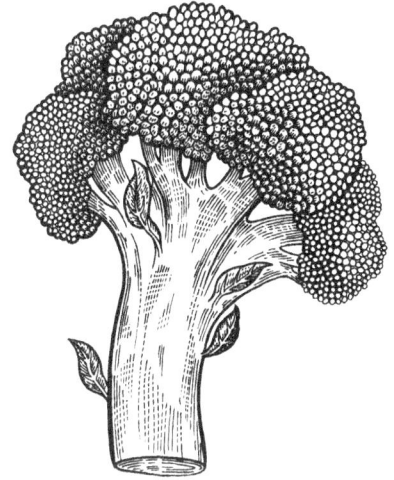

THIS IS HOW YOU MAKE THE RECIPE

1. Wash and trim the ends of the courgette. Make the courgette noodles using a spiralizer and set aside.
2. Heat 1 tablespoon oil in a large pan over medium-high heat. Add the prawns to the hot pan, season with salt and pepper cook for 1 minute.
3. Add the garlic, Italian seasoning, and crushed pepper to the pan. Cook for another minute per side or until the prawns are light pink and garlic is golden brown. Transfer to a bowl.
4. Add the butter and courgette noodles to the same pan, season with salt and pepper and cook for 2 minutes or until tender.
5. Return the cooked prawns to the pan and stir through.
6. Garnished with freshly grated parmesan cheese or/and chopped parsley.

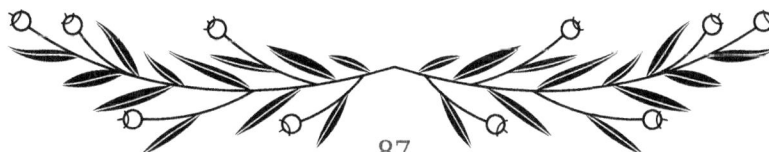

GARLIC STEAK BITES

Servings: 4		Time: 20 min
Nutritional Facts Per Serving:		
Net Carbs:	0.93 g	Protein:	61.5 g
Fat:	41.5 g	Calories:	636 kcal

Ingredients:

100g sirloin steak, cut into 1-inch cubes
1 tbsp olive oil
2 tbsp butter
3-4 garlic cloves, minced or crushed
Salt & black pepper

THIS IS HOW YOU MAKE THE RECIPE

1. Heat oil in a large cast-iron pan for at least 1 minute.
2. Generously season the steak with salt and pepper.
3. Place the steak in the pan in a single layer without overcrowding the pan (work in batches if needed).
4. Cook for 2 minutes per side or until seared and dark brown. Remove the steak from the pan and add the butter and garlic to the pan.
5. Stir for 30 seconds or until the garlic is light brown. Pour garlic over steak bites.
6. Enjoy with some salad (optional).

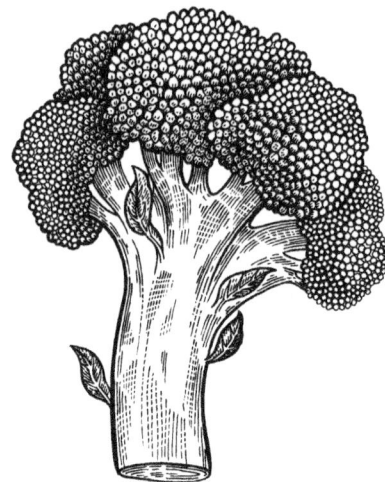

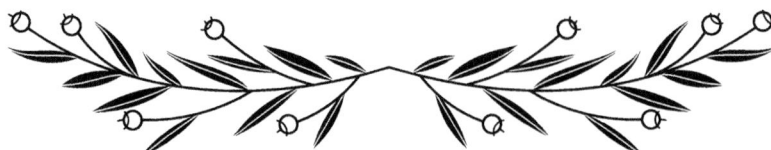

SESAME SALMON, BABY PAK CHOI & MUSHROOMS

Servings: 4   Time: 30 min

Nutritional Facts Per Serving:
Net Carbs: 8 g   Protein: 62 g
Fat: 34.75 g   Calories: 616 kcal

Ingredients:

4 salmon fillets
8 mushrooms
16 baby pak choi
1 tbsp toasted sesame seeds
4 spring onions, chopped

Marinade:
1 tbsp olive oil
1 tsp sesame oil
1 tbsp coconut aminos
1 tsp ginger, grated
1 tsp lemon juice
½ tsp salt
½ tsp black pepper

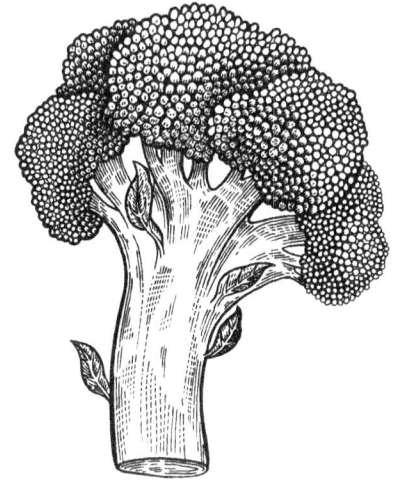

THIS IS HOW YOU MAKE THE RECIPE

1. Whisk all the marinade ingredients together. Drizzle half of the marinade on the salmon and turn to coat.
2. Cover and refrigerate the salmon while it marinates for one hour. Preheat the oven to 200°C.
3. To prepare the vegetables trim the rough ends from the pok choi and cut into halves. Slice the mushrooms into ½-inch pieces. Drizzle the remaining marinade over the vegetables and lay on a lined baking tray.
4. Place salmon, skin side down, on the lined baking tray as well. Bake until salmon is cooked through, about 20 minutes.
5. Top with chopped spring onions and sesame seeds.
6. Serve with grilled or steamed veggies, or a side salad.

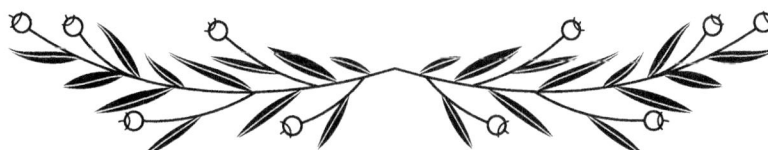

PESTO CHICKEN & VEGGIES

Servings: 4		Time: 25 min
Nutritional Facts Per Serving:		
Net Carbs:	6.47 g	Protein:	37.75 g
Fat:	15 g	Calories:	281 kcal

Ingredients:

4 chicken fillets, chop into bite-size pieces
1-2 cups broccoli florets
1 sweet pepper, chopped
1 large courgette, chopped
¼ cup basil pesto
Optional: ½ cup mozzarella cheese

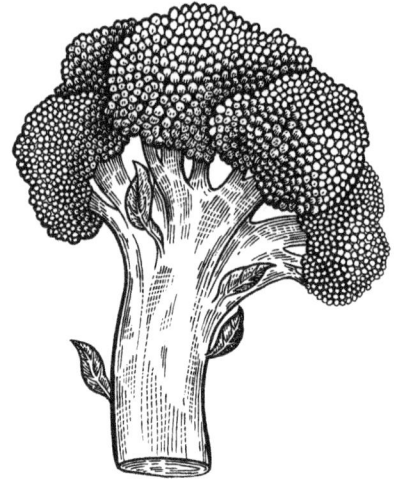

THIS IS HOW YOU MAKE THE RECIPE

1. Pr-heat oven to 218˚C.
2. In a large bowl, combine the chicken, veggies, and pesto until the chicken and veggies are coated well with pesto.
3. Transfer mixture to a large sheet pan and bake for 15-20 minutes.
4. If desired drizzle with mozzarella cheese during the last 5 minutes of baking.
5. Serve and enjoy!

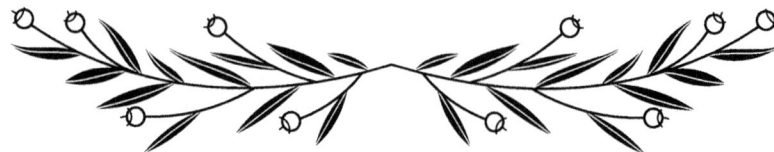

STIR-FRY CHICKEN & VEGGIES

Servings: 4		Time: 20 min
Nutritional Facts Per Serving:		
Net Carbs:	8.56 g	Protein:	35.5 g
Fat:	11 g	Calories:	281 kcal

Ingredients:

2 tbsp olive oil

4 chicken breast fillets, cut into ½-inch slices

2 cups broccoli florets

1 large courgette, cut into slices

1 medium sweet pepper, cut into ½-inch slices

1 medium yellow onion halved & cut into
½-inch slices

½ cup mushrooms

3-4 garlic cloves, minced or crushed

1 tbsp Italian seasoning or your favorite
seasoning

1 tsp salt

½ tsp black pepper

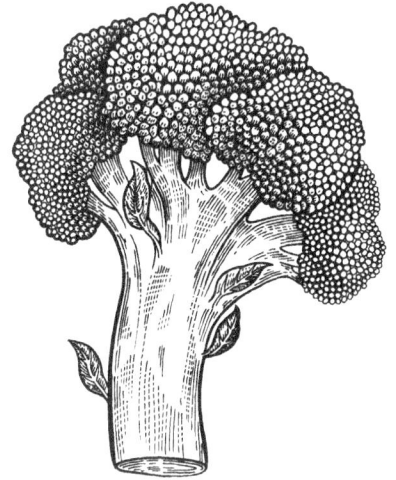

THIS IS HOW YOU MAKE THE RECIPE

1. Heat 2 tablespoons of oil in a large pan to medium-high heat.

2. Add the chicken, veggies, garlic, and spices.

3. Cook for 8-10 minutes, stirring occasionally until the veggies are soft and tender and the chicken is golden and cooked through.

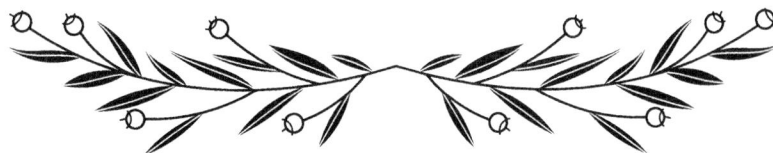

4. Serve and enjoy!

THAI CHICKEN SOUP

Servings: 3		Time: 35 min	
Nutritional Facts Per Serving:			
Net Carbs:	3 g	Protein:	26 g
Fat:	11 g	Calories:	220 kcal

Ingredients:

2 large chicken breasts
½ cup unsweetened coconut milk
½ cup chicken broth
2 cups water
2 tbsp Red Boat fish sauce
1 tbsp Thai garlic chili paste
1 tsp coconut aminos
1 tsp lime juice
½ tsp ginger, ground
1 sprig fresh Thai basil
Coriander to garnish

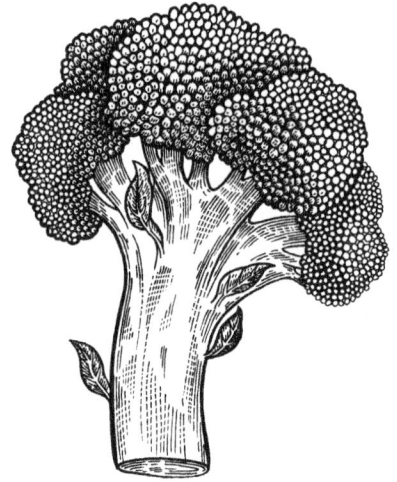

THIS IS HOW YOU MAKE THE RECIPE

1. Thinly slice chicken breasts into ¼-inch thick strips, then cut once more to make the pieces of chicken bite-sized.
2. In a large stock pot, combine coconut milk, broth, water, fish sauce, chili sauce, coconut aminos, lime juice, ginger, and basil.
3. Bring to a boil over high heat.
4. Stir in chicken pieces, reduce heat to low-medium, and cover pot; simmer for 30 minutes.
5. Remove basil leaves from the soup and garnish with coriander.
6. Serve and enjoy!

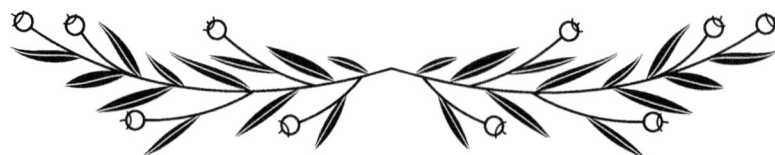

LEMON GARLIC STEAK

Servings: 4		Time: 11 min
Nutritional Facts Per Serving:		
Net Carbs:	2.2 g	Protein:	127 g
Fat:	90 g	Calories:	1327 kcal

Ingredients:

4 (½-inch) top blade steaks
1 tsp salt
½ tsp black pepper
2 tbsp unsalted butter
1 tbsp olive oil
4 garlic cloves, 2 diced & 2 whole
1 lemon's juice
4 asparagus, washed & trimmed

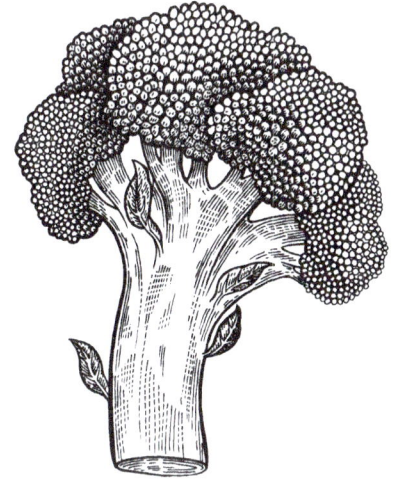

THIS IS HOW YOU MAKE THE RECIPE

1. Pat steaks dry and sprinkle both sides with salt, pepper, diced garlic and a squeeze of lemon.
2. Heat 1 tablespoon butter, olive oil and garlic in a 12-inch heavy pan over moderately high heat until hot but not smoking.
3. Add steaks then sauté 2-3 minutes per side.
4. Squeeze more lemon juice on the steak right before removing from heat.
5. Cook the asparagus until tender and serve with your steak.

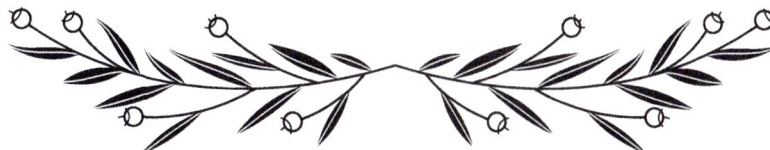

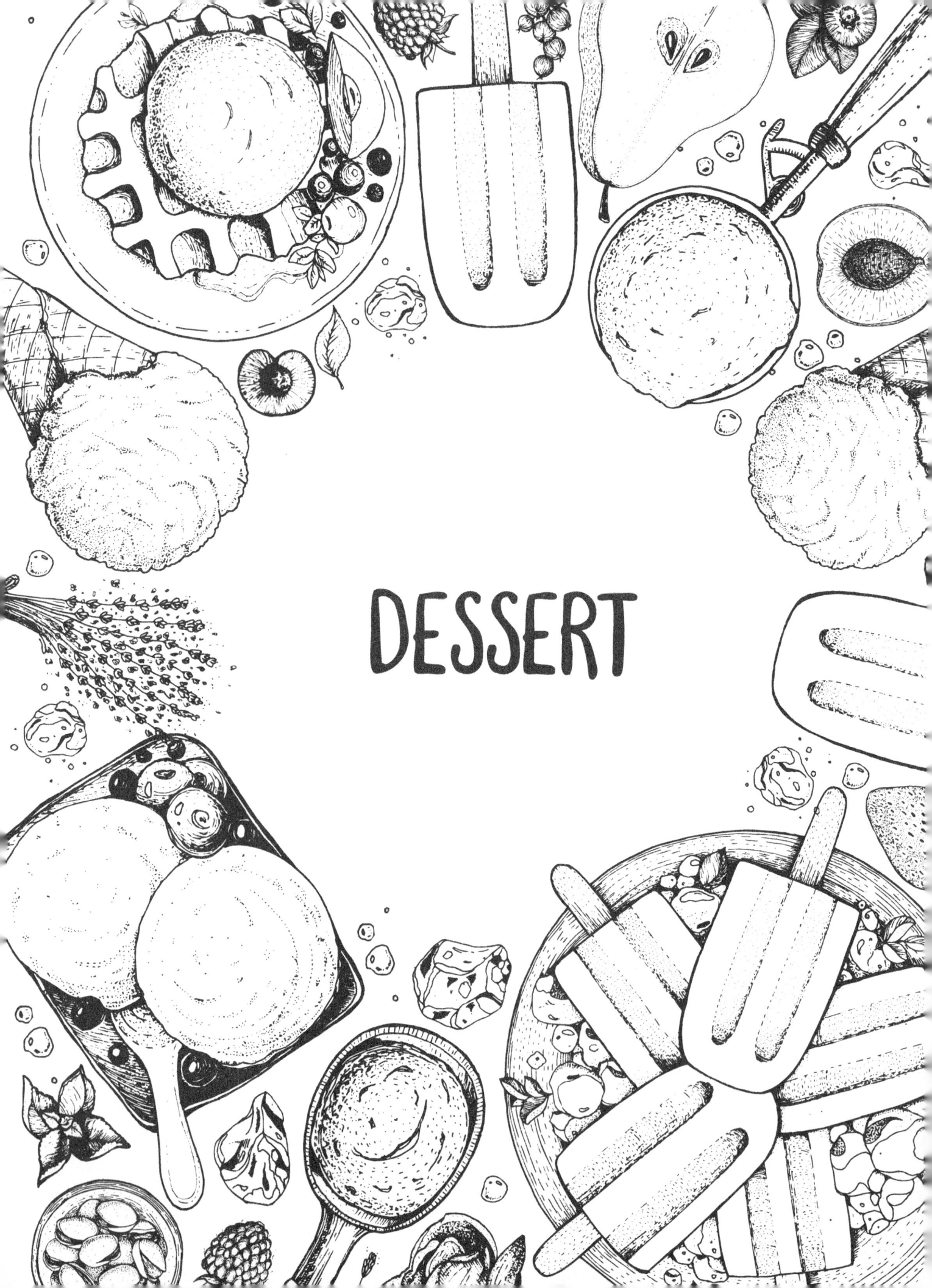

DESSERT

DESSERT MENU

Peanut Butter Fluff Fat Bomb - 96

Chocolate Mousse - 97

Chocolate Peanut Butter Bark - 98

Raspberry Almond Chocolate Fat Bomb Bark - 99

Chocolate Coconut Almond Fat Bombs - 100

PEANUT BUTTER FLUFF FAT BOMB

Servings: 6

Nutritional Facts Per Serving:
Net Carbs: 1.9 g   Protein: 3.8 g
Fat: 14.5 g   Calories: 151 kcal

Ingredients:

½ cup whipping cream
½ soft white cheese (cream cheese, softened)
2¼ tbsp unsweetened peanut butter
5 tbsp Swerve confectioners or Monk Fruit powdered
½ tsp vanilla extract
½ square baking chocolate

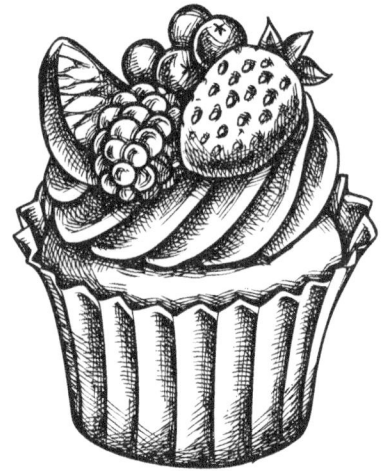

THIS IS HOW YOU MAKE THE RECIPE

1. In a medium-sized bowl, beat whipping cream until it almost doubles in size.
2. In a separate bowl add the softened cream cheese, peanut butter, Swerve confectioners/ Monk Fruit powdered, and vanilla then beat with a mixer until it's smooth and creamy.
3. Combine the two and mix on low until thoroughly combined and smooth.
4. Grate unsweetened chocolate shavings on top.
5. Best kept in the refrigerator overnight and served the next day.

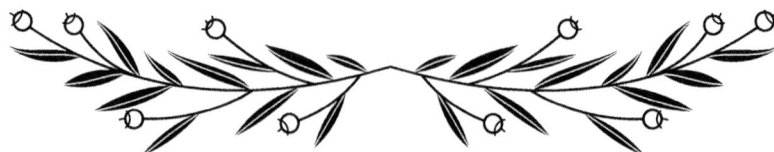

CHOCOLATE MOUSSE

Servings: 4

Nutritional Facts Per Serving:

Net Carbs:	3 g	Protein:	3 g
Fat:	24 g	Calories:	227 kcal

Ingredients:

4 tbsp unsalted butter

4 tbsp soft white cheese (cream cheese)

¼ cup whipping cream

1 tbsp cocoa powder

Stevia, to taste

Optional: 1 tsp coconut oil/MCT oil

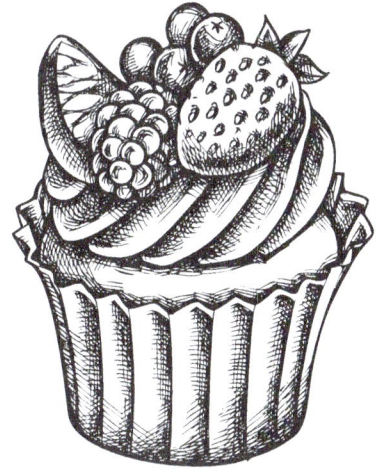

THIS IS HOW YOU MAKE THE RECIPE

1. Soften the butter and combine with sweetener, stirring until completely blended.
2. Add cream cheese and blend until smooth.
3. Add cocoa powder and blend completely.
4. Whip the cream and gradually add to the mixture.
5. If you would like to add more fat, add 1 teaspoon of coconut oil or MCT oil.
5. Spoon into small glasses and refrigerate for 30 minutes.

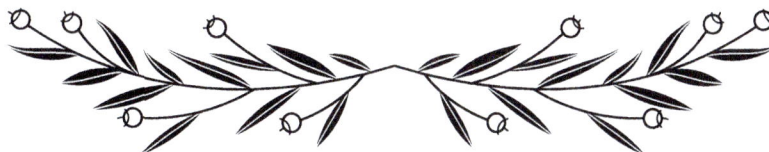

CHOCOLATE PEANUT BUTTER BARK

Servings: 25   Time: 1 h

Nutritional Facts Per Serving:

Net Carbs:	1 g	Protein:	5 g
Fat:	10 g	Calories:	85 kcal

Ingredients:

1 cup coconut oil

¼ cup unsweetened cocoa powder

½ cup natural peanut butter

½ cup sweetener

¼ tsp salt

1 tsp vanilla extract

1 tsp almond extract

½ cup unsweetened coconut flakes

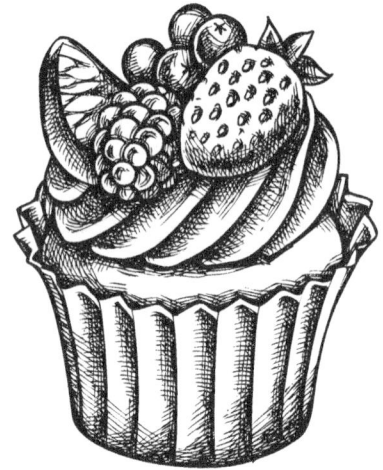

THIS IS HOW YOU MAKE THE RECIPE

1. Melt the coconut oil and peanut butter. Stir until creamy and no chunks of coconut oil remain.
2. Add the salt, sweetener, shredded coconut, almond extract, vanilla extract, and cocoa powder.
3. Mix well.
4. Line a baking tray with greaseproof paper.
5. Pour the melted chocolate onto the greaseproof paper and freeze the chocolate for 45 minutes.
6. Break into pieces & store in a closed container in the freezer.
7. Enjoy!

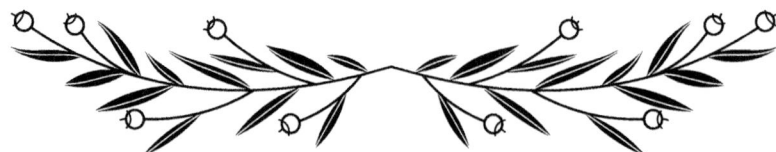

RASPBERRY ALMOND CHOCOLATE FAT BOMB BARK

Servings: 8   Time: 1 h 5 min

Nutritional Facts Per Serving:
Net Carbs: 2.7 g   Protein: 3.09 g
Fat: 7.26 g   Calories: 82 kcal

Ingredients:

¼ cup natural almond butter
½ cup coconut butter
1 tbsp unsweetened cocoa powder
¼ tsp sweetener
⅛ cup raw almonds
⅛ cup walnuts
¼ cup raspberries

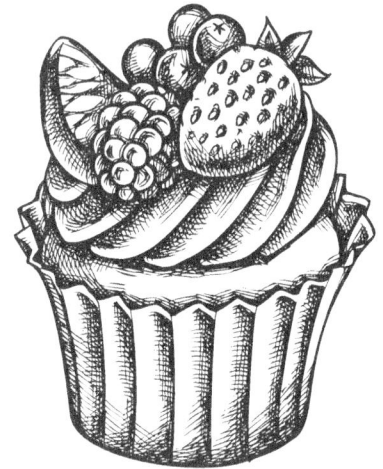

THIS IS HOW YOU MAKE THE RECIPE

1. In a bowl, mix together the coconut butter, almond butter, sweetener and cocoa powder.
2. Chop the almonds and walnuts.
3. Microwave the raspberries for 40-60 seconds and mix.
4. Place some greaseproof paper over a square pan and pour the chocolate butter inside.
5. Sprinkle the nuts over and cover with the melted raspberries.
6. Place in the freezer for 1 hour to freeze. Take it out and break it into 8 pieces (or more if you want smaller portions).
7. Always keep frozen and enjoy!

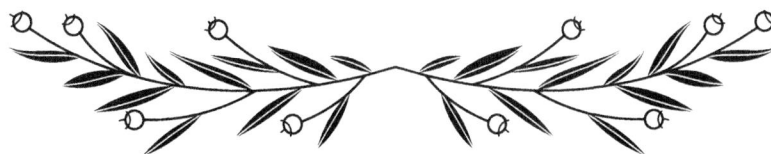

CHOCOLATE COCONUT ALMOND FAT BOMBS

Servings: 30   Time: 1 h 10 min

Nutritional Facts Per Serving:
Net Carbs: 1 g   Protein: 0 g
Fat: 7 g   Calories: 72 kcal

Ingredients:

½ cup coconut oil, melted
½ cup coconut butter/manna, melted
¼ cup unsweetened cocoa powder
1 tsp almond extract
½ tsp vanilla extract
10 drops Stevia or ½ tsp sweetener
¼ cup almonds, crushed slivered
¼ cup unsweetened coconut flakes
¼ cup cacao nibs

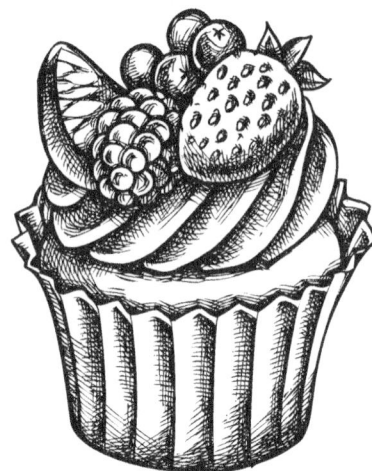

THIS IS HOW YOU MAKE THE RECIPE

1. Mix coconut oil, coconut butter, cocoa powder, almond extract, vanilla extract, and Stevia or sweetener together. If using sweetener: heat in the microwave or on stove for 1-2 minutes until it's dissolved. You may want to taste to check that there are no crunchy crystals.
2. Add in crushed slivered almonds, coconut flakes, and cacao nibs.
3. With a tablespoon, fill mini cupcake liners, mold or an ice cube tray, putting 1 tablespoonful in each.
4. Store in the fridge and enjoy!

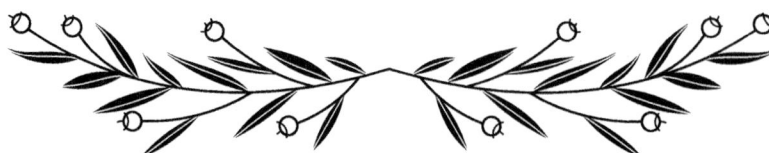

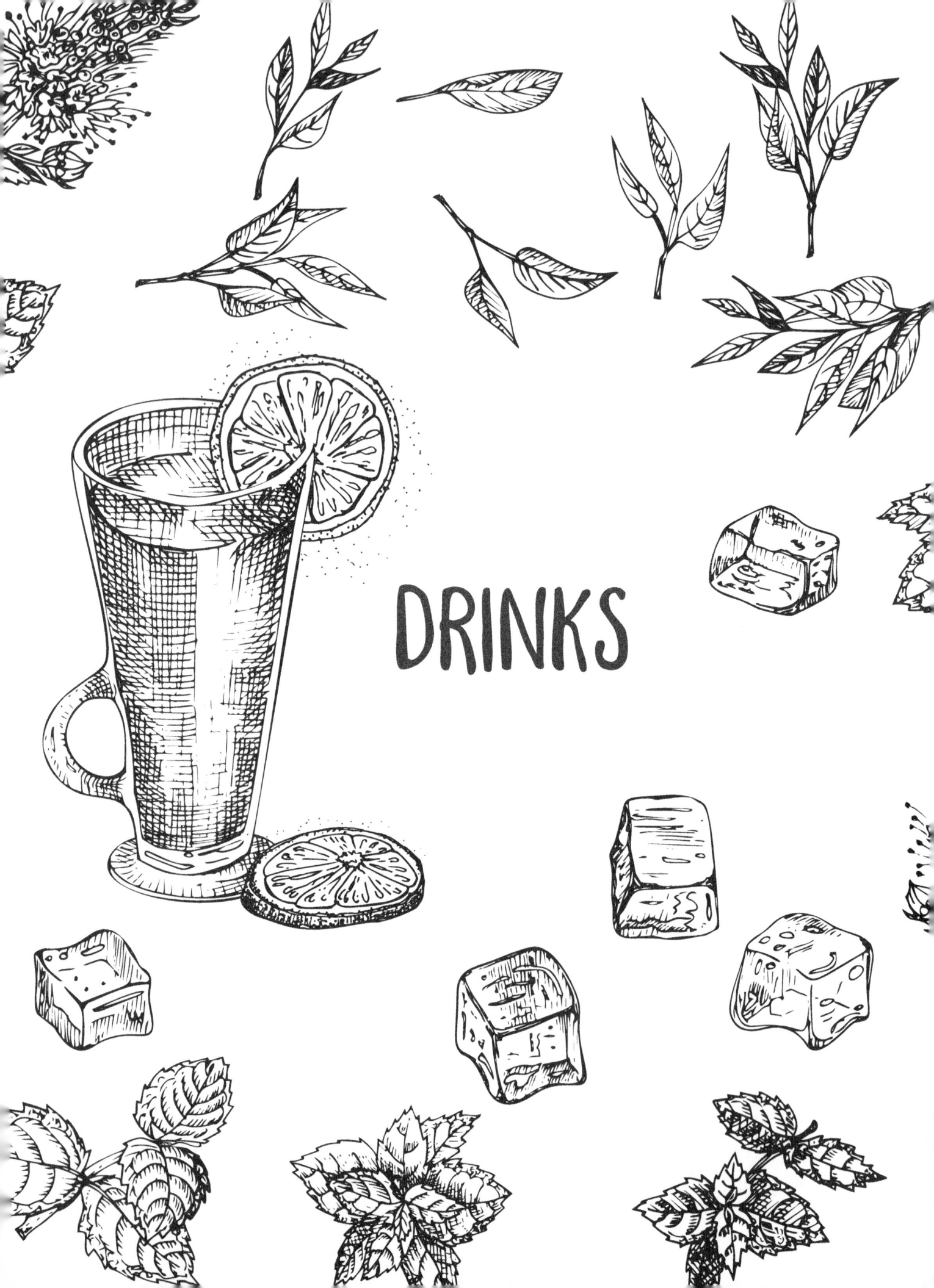

DRINKS

DRINKS MENU

Hot Buttery Coffee - 103

Iced Tea - 104

Flavoured Water - 105

Pumpkin Spice Latte - 106

Hot Chocolate - 107

HOT BUTTERY COFFEE

Ingredients:

1 cup hot coffee, freshly brewed
2 tbsp unsalted butter
1 tbsp MCT oil or coconut oil

THIS IS HOW YOU MAKE THE RECIPE

1. Combine all ingredients in a blender.
2. Blend until smooth and frothy.
3. Serve immediately and enjoy!

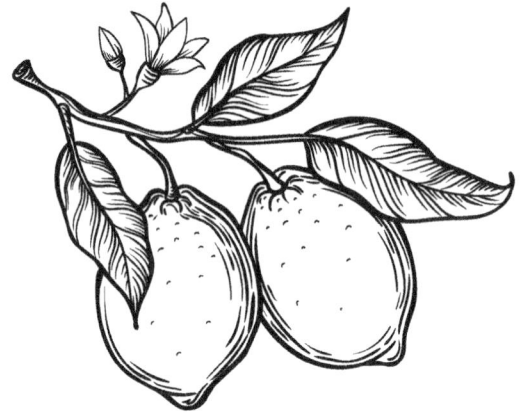

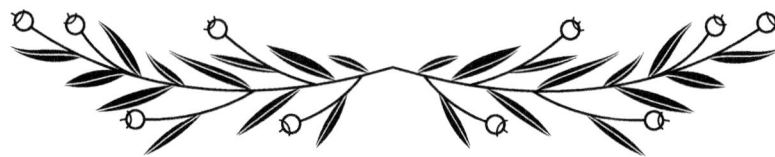

ICED TEA

Servings: 2			
Nutritional Facts Per Serving:			
Net Carbs:	0 g	Protein:	0 g
Fat:	0 g	Calories:	0 kcal

Ingredients:

2 cups cold water
1 tea bag of your choice
1 cup ice cubes
Flavour of your choice: lemon/cucumber/
raspberries/fresh mint

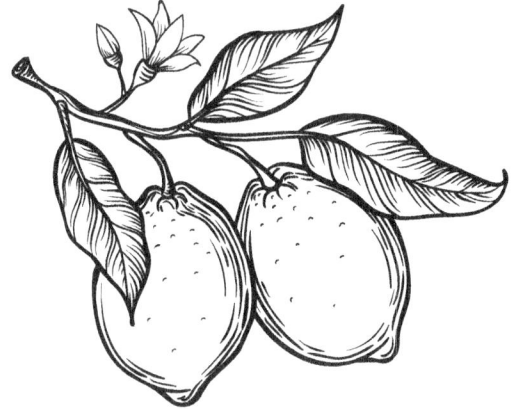

THIS IS HOW YOU MAKE THE RECIPE

1. Combine the tea, flavour of your choice and
half of the cold water in a pitcher.
2. Leave it in the refrigerator for 1-2 hours.
3. Remove the tea bag and the flavouring.
4. Replace with new, fresh flavouring if you so
desire.
5. Add the rest of the cold water and serve with
lots of ice cubes.

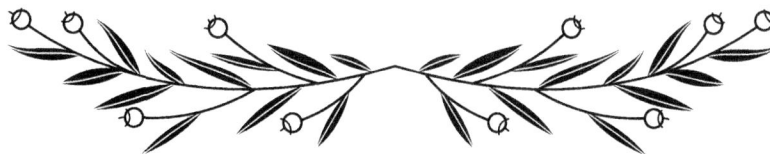

FLAVORED WATER

Servings: 2

Nutritional Facts Per Serving:
Net Carbs: 0 g   Protein: 0 g
Fat: 0 g   Calories: 0 kcal

Ingredients:

4 cups cold water
Flavour of your choice: raspberries/fresh mint/
cucumber/lemon
2 cups ice cubes

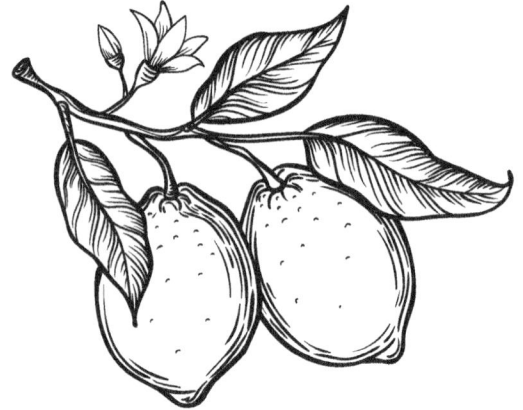

THIS IS HOW YOU MAKE THE RECIPE

1. Pour fresh, cold water into a pitcher.
2. Add Flavour of your choice (berries/mint/
citrus/cucumber/ginger) and refrigerate for 30
minutes.
3. Serve and enjoy!

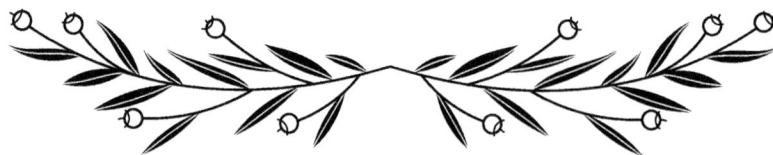

PUMPKIN SPICE LATTE

Servings: 1

Nutritional Facts Per Serving:
Net Carbs: 1 g   Protein: 1 g
Fat: 23 g   Calories: 216 kcal

Ingredients:

2 tbsp unsalted butter
1 tsp pumpkin pie spice/cinnamon
1-2 tsp instant coffee powder
1 cup boiling water
Optional: whipped double cream

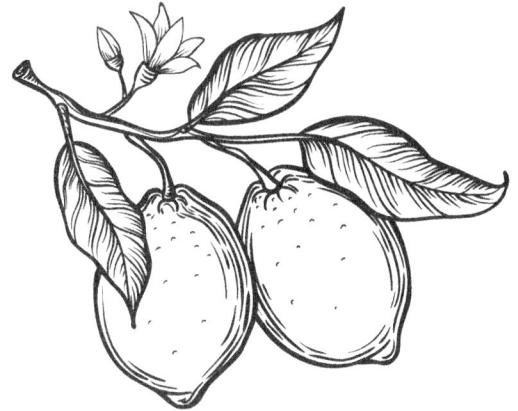

THIS IS HOW YOU MAKE THE RECIPE

1. Place butter, spices and instant coffee (shot of espresso or even decaf) in a deep bowl to use with an immersion blender or blend with a blender.
2. Add boiling water and blend for 20–30 seconds until a fine foam has formed.
3. Pour into a cup and sprinkle some cinnamon or pumpkin spice on top.
4. Optional: Add a scoop of whipped double cream on top and enjoy!

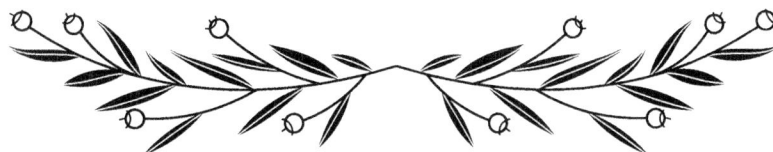

HOT CHOCOLATE

Servings: 1			
Nutritional Facts Per Serving:			
Net Carbs:	1 g	Protein:	1 g
Fat:	23 g	Calories:	216 kcal

Ingredients:

2 tbsp unsalted butter

1 tbsp unsweetened cocoa powder

Optional: 1 tsp powdered sweetener

¼ tsp vanilla extract

1 cup boiling water

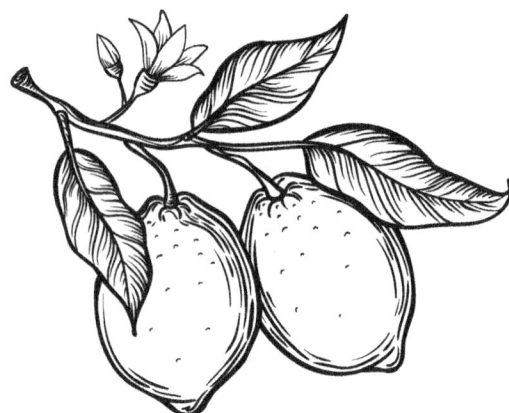

THIS IS HOW YOU MAKE THE RECIPE

1. Put the ingredients in a tall beaker to use with an immersion blender.

2. Mix for 15–20 seconds or until there's a fine foam on top.

3. Pour the hot cocoa into cups and enjoy.

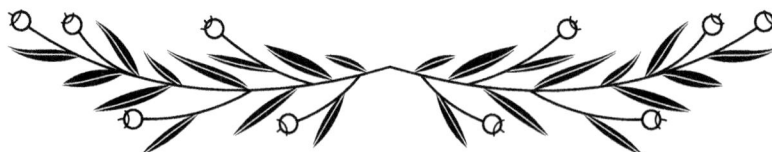

RECOMMENDATIONS FOR IDEAL INGREDIENTS

1. For your molds, get one or more molds or mini muffin pans of different sizes. Molds come with as few as 6 cups and as many as 24.

2. Try to use organic ingredients.

3. Grass-fed/pasture-raised dairy products.

4. Himalayan or sea salt.

5. Spring or filtered water.

6. Fresh herbs.

7. Wash your greens and vegetables before cooking.

8. Use baking chocolate which is 100% dark chocolate or use stevia sweetened dark chocolate.

9. Sweeteners: Monk fruit is the best for the confections and chocolates. Though Swerve, erythritol, stevia and xylitol are all good sweeteners. Never use synthet ic sweeteners!

10. Confectioners' sweeteners: Powdered monk fruit, confectioners' Swerve, or powder your own erythritol or xylitol in a coffee grinder.

11. Use sugar-free or unsweetened ingredients if not otherwise specified.

12. Coconut milk in a tin rather than powdered coconut milk. Also make sure to use the full-fat type.

13. Cooking oil: Avocado oil - it has the highest smoke point.

With the use of the Ketoveo shopping list provided you can put together some yummy ideas of what you would like to eat for your future meal planning.

Remember high fat, moderate protein & low-carbs.

The goal of being on the keto diet is to get your body into a state of ketosis, which means your body is producing ketones (small fuel molecules) from burning fat and not from burning sugar and carbs to create energy for your body.

Ketones are produced when you are eating minimum carbs and moderate protein. This then takes the fats you eat and converts it into ketones by your liver that enter the bloodstream. These ketones are then used as fuel by the cells in the body. They even happily fuel your brain! People feel more energized and focused when the brain runs on ketones, made from fat. This certainly speeds up fat loss being on a ketogenic diet with your body running on your fat as energy!

Following the Ketoveo meal plan can help you on your journey and lifestyle to getting your body healthy, energized and losing weight by getting your body into ketosis.

We wish you the best of luck on your keto journey and we look forward to hearing about your success!

GLOSSARY

Alzheimer's Disease: A disease of the brain that causes people to slowly lose their memory and mental abilities.

Antioxidants: Substances produced by the body and found in foods which defend your body from damage caused by harmful forms of oxygen molecules called free-radicals.

Autism: A condition that begins in childhood that causes problems in forming relationships and in communicating with other people.

Calorie: A unit of food energy.

Carbohydrates: Any one of various substances in food (sugars, starches and fibers found in fruits, grains, vegetables and milk products) that are commonly used as fuel for your body to produce heat and energy.

Diabetes: A serious disease in which the body cannot properly control the amount of sugar in the blood because it does not produce enough insulin; a hormone produced by the Pancreas.

Diet: A controlled regimen of the type and amount of food that a person eats for a certain reason, such as to improve health or to lose weight.

Fat: Fat is a source of fuel; for energy to run the body, and for the process to maintain health. When fat is produced by the body that is not immediately needed, the body stores the fat for future use and energy.

Fatty acids: These are very high-energy fuels. Fatty acids are the building blocks of the fat in our bodies. When the body needs to use the fat as a fuel, it breaks the fat back down into fatty-acids which can then be absorbed into the blood.

Free radicals: Molecules that are highly reactive forms of oxygen which can damage cells. It is believed that having too many free radicals in the body accelerates the progression of cancer, cardiovascular disease, and age-related diseases.

Glucose: Simple sugars the body produces from carbohydrates which the body uses as a fuel. Glucose is preferred by the body as it can use this quicker and easier than fat. When the body produces more glucose than it needs, it converts it to Glycogen and stores it.

Glycogen: A compound made up of many glucose molecules which are then stored in muscles and the liver for later use as fuel. The body can only store a limited amount of glycogen so when it produces too much, the body converts it to fat. All the glycogen stored in the body will be burned up in one day of fasting.

Hayflick limit: When a cell divides, it makes new cells. A cell divides again and again until it reaches the Hayflick limit, usually about fifty and seventy divisions, and then the cell dies.

IGF-1: This is an abbreviation that stands for Insulin-like Growth Factor #1. IGF-1 is a protein made by the liver that stimulates the growth of many types of cells and is similar to insulin. Intermittent fasting on the Keto Diet controls the production of IGF-1.

Inflammation: The body's reaction to injury or infection. The five common signs of inflammation are heat, pain, redness, swelling, and loss of function in the area affected.

Insulin: A hormone that lowers the level of glucose in the blood. It is released into the blood when the glucose level goes up, such as after eating. Insulin helps glucose enter the body's cells, where it can be used for energy or stored for future use.

Ketogenic diet: A diet high in fat, low in carbohydrates (sugars) and an adequate amount of protein. The diet forces the body take fat and convert it to ketones which then become the fuel your body uses to power the body.

Ketosis: A normal metabolic process that takes place when the body does not have glucose to use as its source of energy. When a body is "in ketosis", it uses fat as its primary fuel.

Ketones: When the body breaks down fat into fatty acids, it then breaks down the fatty acids into ketones. Ketones are used by the mitochondria in the cell to become energy for the brain, heart and muscles.

Keto Flu: A collection of symptoms experienced by some people when they first start the keto diet. These symptoms, which can feel similar to the flu, are caused by the body adapting to a new diet consisting of very little carbohydrates.

Liver: A large organ of the body that produces bile and cleans the blood. The liver is one of the largest organs in the body. It has many important functions. It converts the nutrients from food into chemicals the body can use. It stores these substances and supplies cells with them when needed.

Medium-chain triglycerides (MCTs): Triglycerides are the major form of fat in the body. They come from the food we eat as well as from being made by the body. MCTs produce more ketones per unit of energy than normal dietary fats. They influence a feeling of fullness and prevent hunger pangs. Rich food sources of MCTs include coconut oil, palm kernel oil, and dairy products.

Mitochondria: These are tiny "organs" inside the cells which produce the energy the body needs to function. 70% of the energy produced by mitochondria is used by the brain. Cells contain from 1000 to 2500 mitochondria.

Omega-3: A type of fatty acid that lowers cholesterol in the blood, protects against late age-related eye disease and is good for your heart. It is found in salmon and other fish as well as in green leafy vegetables, and some nuts.

Omega-6: A type of fatty acid that lowers cholesterol and reduces the risk of heart disease. A body needs to have it but cannot produce it by itself. Omega-6 fatty acids come from many vegetable oils, nuts, beans, seeds and grains.

Oxidative stress: An imbalance between the production of free radicals and the ability of the body to defend against their harmful effects. Oxidative stress can destroy cells and increase the risk of cancer.

Pancreas: A large gland of the body that is behind the stomach and that produces insulin and other substances that help the body digest food.

Protein: A nutrient found in foods such as meat, milk, eggs, and beans that is a necessary part of the diet and is essential for normal cell structure, muscle and function. Sebum: Is an oily substance produced by glands in your skin which act as a lubricant for the hair and skin. It also provides some protection against bacteria and helps preserve the flexibility of the hair.

Starch: A carbohydrate that is found in certain foods, such as bread, rice, and potatoes. The body turns starch into glucose for use as fuel.

Sugar: A sweet substance especially from the plants sugar cane and sugar beet, used to make food and drinks sweet. The body turns sugar into glucose for use as a fuel.

Printed in Great Britain
by Amazon